THE CHEMISTRY AND MATHEMATICS OF DNA POLYHEDRA

DNA: PROPERTIES AND MODIFICATIONS, FUNCTIONS AND INTERACTIONS, RECOMBINATION AND APPLICATIONS

DNA: Fingerprinting, Sequencing and Chips
Kresten Ovesen and Ulrich Matthiesen (Editors)
2009. 978-1-60741-814-6

DNA Adducts: Formation, Detection and Mutagenesis
Emerson Álvarez and Roberto Cunha (Editors)
2010. 978-1-60741-433-9

Sperm Nuclear Maturation: A Basic and Clinical Approach
Ali Reza Talebi
2010. 978-1-61668-194-4

The Chemistry and Mathematics of DNA Polyhedra
Wen-Yuan Qiu, Ze Wang, and Guang Hu
2010. 978-1-61668-589-8

The Chemistry and Mathematics of DNA Polyhedra
Wen-Yuan Qiu, Ze Wang, and Guang Hu
2010. 978-1-61668-296-5

Sperm Nuclear Maturation: A Basic and Clinical Approach
Ali Reza Talebi
2010. 978-1-61668-495-2

DNA: PROPERTIES AND MODIFICATIONS, FUNCTIONS
AND INTERACTIONS, RECOMBINATION AND APPLICATIONS

THE CHEMISTRY AND MATHEMATICS OF DNA POLYHEDRA

WEN-YUAN QIU,
ZE WANG
AND
GUANG HU

Nova Science Publishers, Inc.
New York

LIBRARY OF CONGRESS CATALOGING-IN-PUBLICATION DATA
Available upon Request

ISBN: 978-1-61668-296-5

Published by Nova Science Publishers, Inc. ✛ New York

CONTENTS

PREFACE

Polyhedra have attracted scientists' attentions due to their high-symmetric architectures since ancient times, and even served as common modes in natural world, for example, the polyhedral skeletons of molecular structures. Chemists, in the past few centuries, have strived to synthesize these polyhedral targets. Despite achievements that have been arrived, there is still a gap between the great varieties of polyhedral shapes observed in nature (such as viral protein capsids) and the relatively limited molecular polyhedra constructed by small organic molecules. Fortunately, DNA was shown to be an excellent material in molecular construction. The construction of polyhedral structures with DNA improves the development of synthetic chemistry, and meanwhile, produces some complicated molecules with novel topological and geometrical structures, such as the DNA tetrahedron, DNA cube, DNA octahedron, DNA dodecahedron, and DNA icosahedron, as well as the tetrahedral DNA cage and the hexahedral DNA box, and so on. Interests on these novel architectures have inspired mathematical considerations and modeling of a new theory of polyhedra, including structure construction, symmetry analysis, chirality detection and invariant calculation. Herein, we have summarized advances in the chemical syntheses of DNA polyhedra, which also have been envisaged and classified by underlying principles of geometry and symmetry. Moreover, this paper reviews our recent progresses in the theoretical investigation of a new mathematical theory of DNA polyhedra.

Chapter 1

1. INTRODUCTION

Once the great geometer Coxeter wrote: '…the chief reason for studying regular polyhedra is still the same as in the times of the Pythagoreans, namely, that their symmetrical shapes appeal to one's artistic sense'.[1] These beautiful objects attract continuously consideration and discussion of mathematicians from ancient times, writing them as one of the oldest chapters in mathematics; and arise the interests of artists, architects and philosophers, making them as an icon of human civilization.[2] Meanwhile, these symmetric structures are also favored in the laboratory and nature.[2, 3] Chemists, molecular architects, fascinated by these symmetrical molecular structures, have been making great efforts in synthesizing these beautiful molecules, by chemically constructing the Platonic solids such as tetrahedron, cube, dodecahedron with small organic molecules and other polyhedra from supermolecular self-assembly.[3-9] The preference for highly symmetric objects with a spherical shape is also found in the case of life, such as the icosahedral shape of a viral capsid protein, the polyhedral structure of Clathrin protein and the cuboctahedral structure of the COPII protein, for examples.[10-16] These endeavors would enlarge and improve our knowledge and skills on synthetic chemistry, and moreover, bring new insights into ubiquitous polyhedral structures of molecules in nature. On the other hand, chemical syntheses of these elegant molecules and their underlying biological complexity have been turned out to be of great challenges.

Fortunately, the life molecule DNA, with amazing abilities, could be utilized as a fantastic material in constructing polyhedral structures.[17, 18] Such a groundbreaking idea, synthesizing polyhedra with genetic material DNA, was first proposed by Ned Seeman and even hoped to fabricate regular

3D architectures extending into 3-space at the very beginning.[19, 20] In practice, this magic molecule really performs amazing self-assembly and programmable abilities in laboratories.[17, 18] During the past two decades, chemists have created a series of polyhedral molecules, far more complicated and delicate than ever before.[21-25] These fulfillments open the door to structural DNA nanotechnology and take chemists a further step towards mimicking nature.[26-33] And now, constructing and synthesizing various polyhedron-shaped molecules is a fast growing area in current chemistry. The DNA nanopolyhedra or DNA nanocages, which use DNA as a building material to synthesize polyhedra with nanometer precision, have strongly evoked the research interests of the prodigious and distinguished group of chemists. Although there is much to probe, the stakes are high and the odds for success are excellent.

A number of interesting problems, on the other hand, on characterization and analysis of polyhedral molecules in the syntheses have been proposed, which are now challenging mathematical theory of the nanopolyhedra. Novel topological structures, interlocked and interlinked due to DNA double helices, emerge from DNA nanopolyhedra, differing them from polyhedra. Detailed background information on several newer results can be found in Refs. [21-25]. It is now clear that this is an area ripe for development and deserves special encouragement. However, a great deal of essential feature of the nanopolyhedra is either unknown or, at best, poorly understood. Therefore, systematic understandings of these curious objects in details need new mathematics. Scientists are now vigorously studying DNA nanopolyhedra architectures and, little by little, piecing together a new branch of mathematics, although the full story has yet to be written. Based on graph theory and knot theory, polyhedral links, a novel mathematical model, have been proposed to phrase and answer their structural characteristics.[34] It is believed that polyhedral links are new forms of polyhedra, which open enormous challenges and opportunities for scientists in at least two disciplines. One is that they are potential targets in synthetic chemistry, and the other is that they might lay chances for development of new theories in mathematics. As we will, now see, nanopolyhedra not only provide a unifying framework for chemistry, but it may well forge an equally deep union with mathematics as well.

2. BUILDING POLYHEDRA WITH DNA

2.1. WHY POLYHEDRA?

Polyhedron is a model of the eyes and the hands as well as of the mind.[35] In fact, connections between polyhedra and chemistry have been established since ancient times.[36] Plato made systematic considerations on relationships between the real material world and the idea of geometry world. He described firstly five regular polyhedra, known as Platonic polyhedra, and imagined that the element fire could be represented by tetrahedron, earth by cube, air by octahedron, water by icosahedron, and the universe by dodecahedron. Later, the idea of representing elements with five Platonic polyhedra was shown to be impractical. However, it did not disturb chemists' constantly exploring polyhedral models for chemical structures of material world. Without respect to the important tetrahedron and octahedron model in stereochemistry, several unexpected complicated polyhedra are proved to be basic molecular structural model. In 1937, mathematician M. Goldberg, when solving isoperimetric problems of polyhedra, discovered a family of complex polyhedra, namely Goldberg polyhedra, which consists of twelve pentagons and certain numbers of hexagons only.[37] Later in the laboratory, one of the exotic complex polyhedra were found to exist as the third allotrope of carbon, buckminsterfullerenes.[38, 39] More surprisingly, Goldberg polyhedra could be even modeled as frameworks of spherical virus capsid, affording a structural classification for viruses.[11, 40]

Interested in molecules of complex polyhedral structures, biological or nonbiological, chemists are making efforts on synthesizing the beautiful structures in laboratory. As progresses it would bring to synthetic chemistry, some new insights into biomacromolecules, such as viral capsids, might also break out as benefits. Undoubtedly, the polyhedral world is nice and alive in all ages, included ours!

2.2. WHEN DNA MEETS POLYHEDRA

As a fundamental material of life, DNA is functioned as the basis of replication and transcription. In 1953, Watson and Crick proposed the famous double helix structure as the molecular model of genetics, which describes DNA as two polymers of nucleotides run in opposite directions with backbones held together by the hydrogen bond between purine and pyrimidine, with the specific interactions as Adenine (A) bonded to Thymine (T) and Cytosine (C) to Guanine (G).[41, 42] These perfect complementarities provide clear molecular pictures of genetic replication, and uncover the powerful molecular self-reorganization and self-assembly ability of DNA. It is the amazing property that makes DNA a wonderful material for nanoconstruction. Moreover, other features such as a persistence length of 50nm under normal conditions,[43] geometric regularity regardless of particular sequences of nucleotides[44] and proper length scale of 2nm in width (B-DNA)[45] are also critical for constructing three-dimensional nano-materials with DNA.[17, 18]

With the help of branched DNA, Seeman [20] proposed that DNA could be reconstructed by modern biotechnology, sticky-ended cohesion technique, into three-dimensional structures. Branched DNA, also DNA junction, differs from DNA of natural configuration, extending not in one but higher dimensions.[46, 47] During the process of genetic recombination, information exchanges between two DNA helices by a branched DNA known as Holliday junction.[48] However, the Holliday junction is mobile that four strands will eventually separate into two new duplexes by sliding, and therefore not suitable for DNA nanoconstruction. In order to stabilize the structure, Seeman proposed that one can break the sequence symmetry of DNA junctions by designing artificial DNA sequences using a computer program.[20, 46, 47] Indeed, he and co-workers obtained a series of immobile DNA junctions with different arms in laboratory, which made the synthesis of DNA polyhedra richer.[49, 50]

With various stable junctions in hand, it is natural to construct three-dimensional structures by synthesizing vertices of certain valence with DNA junctions of appropriate arm numbers and joining these junctions by sticky-ended cohesion further (Figure 1).[20] In early 1990s, Seeman's group made the ground-breaking progress in DNA three-dimensional construction by subtle synthesis of DNA cube and truncated octahedron.[51, 52]

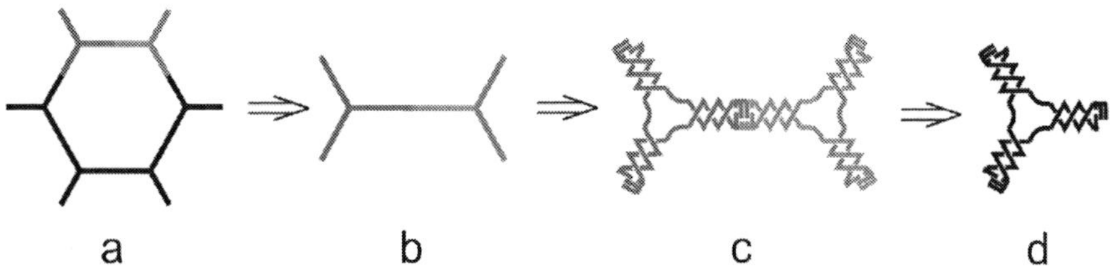

Figure 1. Schematic illustration of the principle of DNA nanoconstruction. Any geometric motifs (a) can be decomposed into the joint of vertices (b), which can be reconstructed with DNA junctions through sticky-ended cohesion (c).

The synthesis of DNA cube and truncated octahedron is step-wise and provides great control at each step during the construction. However, the protocol is time-consuming, of quite low yield and poor rigidity, difficult for asymmetry sequence design, and not replicable. Therefore, chemists later were dedicated to develop strategies of high efficiency, excellent stereoselectivity, good rigidity, and acceptable sequence design task. Over the past 20 years, these strategies have been successfully performed in laboratory by constructing series of DNA polyhedra, providing an effective approach towards mimicking nature and refreshing knowledge and technology of synthetic chemistry![21-25, 33] These represent a tremendous challenge and opportunity for modern chemistry, and for the chemists of the future.

3. DNA POLYHEDRA

3.1. PLATONIC SOLIDS

It has been mathematically proved that there are only five Platonic polyhedra, i.e. tetrahedron, cube, octahedron, dodecahedron, and icosahedron. Each of these solids consists of identical regular faces, and possesses the highest symmetry of all polyhedra (Figure 2a).[2,35]

Point symmetry group analysis shows that the tetrahedron is T_d symmetry, the cube and octahedron are O_h, and the dodecahedron and icosahedron are I_h, respectively. Specifically, without respect to the geometrical and topological structure of DNA helix, the symmetry property of DNA polyhedra is decided exclusively by the symmetric characteristics of DNA sequences on each edge. Therefore, it is convenient to characterize point symmetry group of DNA polyhedra through the analysis of possible symmetry elements of DNA sequences on edges, i.e., 2-fold rotation axis C_2 (palindrome) and reflection mirror σ (Figure 2b). If, by some reasons, the mirror symmetry element σ of DNA sequences was broken, the point group T_d, O_h, I_h of polyhedra will be transformed to T, O, I, respectively. These lower point group (T, O, I) will be degenerated into C_1 (no symmetry) in the case of the absence of rotation axis C_2, which means the DNA sequence is not a palindrome.

The beautiful simplicity of the symmetry principles pursues an inner harmony, where elegance, uniqueness and beauty define molecular structures.

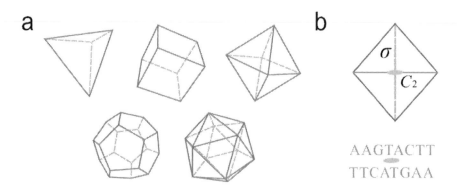

Figure 2. Five Platonic polyhedra. Each is composed of same regular faces, and thus is highly symmetrical.

3.1.1. DNA Tetrahedron

The chemical synthesis of DNA tetrahedron was initiated by Turberfield's group in 2004.[53] With great interests on this molecular tetrahedron, several groups redesigned the synthetic strategy with a number of DNA tetrahedra and their derivatives (Turberfield *et al.*, 2005 [54]; Mao *et al.*, 2008 [55]; Yan *et al.*, 2009 [56,57]; Alivisatos *et al.*, 2009 [58]; Armitage *et al.*, 2009 [59]).

In 2004, Turberfield and colleagues in Oxford reported the synthesis of a DNA tetrahedron, by assembling four appropriately designed oligonucleotides in an annealing process.[53] Each oligonucleotide contains 55 nucleotides (nt), and is consisted of three subsequences of 17 basepairs (bp) hinged by two nucleotides, which are designed to complement uniquely with subsequences of other strands forming DNA duplexes, as edges of a tetrahedron.[53] Four strands were combined with equimolar quantities, and after annealed the system from 95 ℃ to 20 ℃ they obtained the DNA tetrahedra within only about four minutes.[53] The DNA tetrahedron contains four nicks at each vertex where the 3' and 5' ends of an ssDNA meet (Figure 3a). And a couple of stereoisomers may exist due to the different subsequences on each edge.[53] The high-resolution structure of DNA tetrahedron was recently confirmed by Turberfield *et al.* with the help of cryoEM technique. [60]

In the successive experiment, with a few improvements, the group showed the synthesis has very good stereoselectivity.[54] They reduced two hinge nucleotides to one and moved four nicks to edges of tetrahedron. Therefore, the improved DNA tetrahedron differs from the former one, containing two edges of intact DNA double helix, which will form easily in intramolecular reaction. The synthesis produces only one stereoisomer with certain configuration at a vertex with high yield (>95%) in only several seconds, indicating both laudable stereochemical control and efficiency of the strategy.[54]

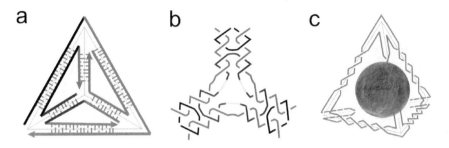

Figure 3. (a) Schematic representations of DNA tetrahedra. DNA subsequences in the same colors are complementary to form edges of tetrahedra.[54] (b) '3-point star' motif developed by Mao et al. [55] to synthesize DNA tetrahedron. Red, green, black colors indicate long, medium and short DNA strands, respectively. Yellow colors in the medial represent three unpaired loops. (c) DNA tetrahedron (orange) that encapsulates a protein (yellow) inside [29].

Based on this strategy, the group synthesized a series of DNA tetrahedra, ones of different edge length,[54] one with a reconfigurable edge,[31] and one with protein molecule encaged (Figure 3c).[29] The geometric structures and parameters of these DNA tetrahedra are summarized in Table 1.

Table 1. Edge parameters of some DNA tetrahedral

DNA tetrahedra	Edge parameters
A series of tetrahedra of different edge lengths	3×20bp/3×30bp; 5×20bp/1×(10,15,20,25,30)bp; 4×20bp/1×10bp/1×(10,15,20,25,30)bp*
Tetrahedron with a reconfigurable edge	5×20bp/1×10bp; 5×20bp/1×30bp
Tetrahedron encapsulating a protein inside	6×20bp

* The notation, for example '4×20bp/1×10bp/1×(10,15,20,25,30)bp' means four edges of tetrahedron contain 20bp, one 10bp, and the left either 10, 15, 20, 25, or 30bp.[29, 53, 54].

The synthetic strategy developed by Turberfield's group combines several strands by self-assembly in a single step process, proceeds with high yield and good stereochemical selectivity, providing a useful method in the synthesis of DNA polyhedra. This is a tremendous achievement, but it is only part of the reason nanopolyhedra have generated such excitement.

Recently, Mao and his fellow researchers reconstructed DNA tetrahedra by an extraordinary effective strategy, which assembles many copies of identical building blocks in a hierarchical fashion.[55] The building block is designed as intermediate tile that self-assembles into final structures in the next step in the hierarchy process.[61-65] The tile '*n*-point star' is a *n*-arm branched structure, which is actually a combination of DNA duplexes connected with several unpaired loops, providing both a better stiffness of the branched arms and a controllable flexibility over the whole motif that could be used in a variety of DNA nanostructures (Figure 3b).[66, 67]

In the synthesis of DNA tetrahedra, '3-point star' was used according to 3-valent vertex of tetrahedra. It consists of a long strand (Figure 3b, red), three identical medium strands (Figure 3b, green), and three identical short strands (Figure 3b, black), forming a 3-fold symmetrical structure.[55] Each of its arms is 21bp in length and 4nm in width, as a pair of DNA double helix joined side by side.[55] Meanwhile, the tile contains three unpaired loops with length variable, making different flexibility possible (Figure 3b, yellow).[55]

In the hierarchical self-assembly process, three types of DNA strands combine first into '3-point star' tiles, and then assemble into DNA tetrahedra. By adjusting the concentration of the tiles (75 nanomolar (nM)) and the length of loops (5nt each), DNA tetrahedron were obtained in a one-pot reaction with a yield of 90%.[55] Each tetrahedron consists of four '3-point star' at vertices, contains 42bp in length per edge.[55]

The hierarchical self-assembly strategy provides an effective way to synthesize DNA polyhedra with high yield. Furthermore, the process involves only identical building blocks, avoiding difficulty of sequences design task.[25, 55]

Most recently, Yan and co-workers [56] constructed a DNA tetrahedral container by self-assembling sheets of scaffolded DNA, which is enclosed by four triangular faces (Figure 4a). Alivisatos *et al.* [58] have successfully assembled gold colloid to four vertices of a DNA tetrahedron (Figure 4b), and Armitage and his research group [59] have prepared fluorescent DNA tetrahedron with tunable wavelength. It is believed that the explorations of constructing DNA tetrahedron will find their powerful applications in the near future. More curiously, Yan and his team [57] have reported the design and construction of a nanometer-sized tetrahedron from a single strand of DNA that is 286 nucleotides long. The potential gains from these exciting results are considerable.

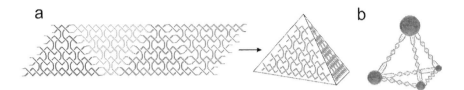

Figure 4. (a) The tetrahedral DNA cage.[56] Self-assembly of 4 DNA triangular sheets (left) into a DNA tetrahedral container (right). Different colors of DNA sheets indicate different triangular faces of DNA tetrahedron. (b) Gold colloid (yellow balls) assembled at each corner of a DNA tetrahedron [58].

Symmetry in nanopolyhedra has a very concrete and precise meaning, and it is a key part of aesthetics. The symmetry of DNA polyhedra differs from geometric polyhedra due to primary structures of DNA sequences on edges, which is referred as molecular symmetry breaking.[68] The molecular symmetry breaking is a mechanism by which a system of itself goes from a high symmetric conformation to a non-symmetric one. We say that some molecules are more symmetric than others are, or that some molecules have high symmetry while others have low symmetry or no symmetry. Most artificial DNAs may have high symmetry or no symmetry, whereas the natural DNAs have no symmetry.

Turberfield synthesized the DNA tetrahedron [53] which contains asymmetric DNA sequences on edges. For example, one of these sequences can be represented as:

$$\frac{\text{ACATTCCTAAGTCTGAA}}{\text{TGTAAGGATTCAGACTT}},$$

where a central line means two single strands (upper and below) are bonded complementarily to form a DNA helix. It can be intuitively seen that the sequence (the helix) is lack of either a reflection mirror σ or a rotation axis C_2, i.e., not a palindrome. As a result, according to the analysis in Section 3.1, the DNA tetrahedron possesses only C_1 symmetry, the least symmetry or in other words, no symmetry. And, it is impossible to recover the symmetry state of DNA tetrahedron by redesigning DNA palindrome sequences because there are odd numbers of bases (17bp) in the sequence. For example, the following redesigned sequence cannot be a palindrome to reserve the C_2 symmetry due to the central paired bases A and T. Obviously, a rotation axis does not exist between these two bases.

ACATTCCTAAGGAATGT
TGTAAGGATTCCTTACA

Thus, the DNA tetrahedron synthesized by Turberfield *et al.* [53] can not possess higher point symmetry group through DNA sequences redesign without changing the number of bases on edges.

On the other hand, the DNA tetrahedron constructed by Mao *et al.* [55] contains parallel DNA helices on each edge, which can be written as follows:

CCTACGATGGACACGGTAACGCCTAGCAACCTGCCTGGCAAG
GGATGCTACC TGTGCCATTGCGGATCGTTGGACGGACCGTTC

CTTGCCAGGCAGGTTGCTAGGCGTTACCGTGTCCATCGTAGG
GAACGGTCCGTCCAACGATCCGCAATGGCACAGGTAGCATCC

According to this representation, it can be easily discovered a rotation axis C_2 exist at the center of these sequences, which ensures that the DNA tetrahedron constructed by Mao *et al.* [55] belongs to the point group *T*. Symmetry analysis tell us, intuitively at least, that two states of the system must differ in their DNA sequences.

3.1.2. DNA Cube

The possibility of synthesizing a cube with DNA was first investigated by Seeman's group in 1991.[51] Later, researchers reconstructed DNA cube with improved techniques (Mao *et al.*, 2009 [69]; Andersen *et al.*, 2009 [70]; Kuzuya *et al.*, 2009 [/1]). Until now, there exist three independent approaches to construct DNA cube. [51, 69, 70]

DNA cube was first synthesized by Seeman's group in 1991 with 3-arm DNA junctions.[51] They first constructed two squares representing a pair of opposite faces of a cube, and then connected them by joining the sticky ends of corresponding vertices.[51] Belt-like intermediate in the reaction might enclose itself in two opposite ways, resulting in a pair of stereoisomers (Figure

5a).[51] The final cube was compose of six DNA strands, intertwining together to form an interesting molecular catenane with novel topology.[72] Each edge of the cube contains 20bp, 6.8nm, i.e. two helical turns (Figure 5b).[51]

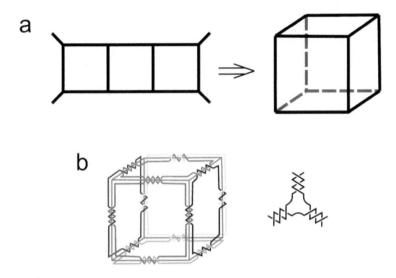

Figure 5. Synthesis of DNA cube. (a) DNA cube (right) can be reconstructed from belt-like intermediate (left). Enclosure of the intermediate, insides and outsides, will produce two different isomers. (b) The catenaned structure of DNA cube (right) and 3-armed DNA junction used in the synthesis (left). DNA cube is consisted of six different strands, each running around a face of the cube [51].

As a milestone, the synthesis of DNA cube opens the door of DNA nanotechnology and provides the fundamental strategy in DNA nanoconstruction by fabricating 3D objects by joining each DNA junction together. However, the protocol is step-wise, time-consuming, and proceeds with quite low yield. Therefore, chemists later were dedicated to develop strategies of high efficiency.

DNA cube was rebuilt recently by Mao *et al.* by self-assembly of '3-point star' motifs.[69] Different from the synthesis of DNA tetrahedra, two types of motifs are used as building units in the manner that different motifs A and B are linked whereas same motifs are not.[69] Consequently, the geometrical objects constructed must contain even number of vertices on each face in order to form a closed structure.[69] Obviously, cube is the smallest and simplest one in this class. So, it can be formed first at low concentration.[69]

Mao's group [69] designed two complementary ways to assemble two types of motifs into a cube. One way is to design two completely different types of '3-point star' motifs consisted of same backbones but different DNA sequences, so that DNA sequences at the sticky-ends of motifs are complementary only among the different types.[69] As a result, one type of motifs can bind only to another different type rather than the same.[69] In other words, association between different types of motifs, say type A and B, is possible, whereas interactions between same types, A-A or B-B, is impossible. Using the idea, they constructed DNA cube with two types of motifs, each containing 5nt unpaired loop and of concentration 200nM.[69] The DNA cube consists of two completely different types of motifs arranged alternatively at vertices, two DNA double helices on each edge, each of 42bp, 4 turns (Figure 6 above).[69]

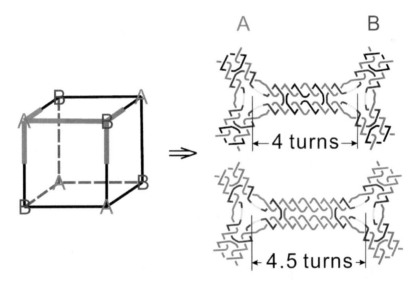

Figure 6. Schematic illustration of the synthesis of DNA cube with '3-point star' motif. DNA cube (left) can be built with two different types of motifs in the manner that different motifs A and B are linked whereas same motifs are not. Mao *et al.* designed the two motifs A and B by two complementary approaches, either by using two completely different types of '3-point star' motifs consisted of same backbones but different DNA sequences (left, above) or by connecting two motifs of same sequences but with different face orientations (left, below) [69].

Except for the straightforward method, another strategy was designed as a complementary way. It is more subtle in that two types of motifs are actually composed of identical DNA sequences. However, two different interactions come out on the consideration of two opposite faces of '3-point star' motifs.[69] The faces of two motifs linked through DNA helices will be on opposite sides if the helix is odd numbers of half-turns, and vice versa.[62] And thus, two different sides of '3-point star' are connected alternatively as two different types of motifs. Therefore, they designed the helices of each edge to be 4.5 turns rather than 4 turns usually involved.[62, 69] By controlling the concentration to be 50nM and unpaired loop of 5nt, DNA cubes were obtained in the hierarchical self-assembly process of a single type of '3-point star'.[69] Different from the former one, the cube contains 47bp on each DNA helical edge, that is, 4.5 helical turns (Figure 6, below).[62, 69]

In general, the method developed in the synthesis of DNA cube with two types of tiles makes good control at the face geometry of DNA polyhedra in that only the one with even number of vertices on each face can be possibly produced.[69] Consequently, it complements the strategy of hierarchical self-assembly, and thus benefits DNA polyhedra construction.[69] But even this is not quite the end of the story.

Very recently, based on the idea of single stranded DNA origami, Andersen and co-workers have constructed a DNA cube enclosed by six DNA sheets (Figure 7).[70] This DNA box, with 42×36×36 nm3 in size, can be utilized as a DNA nanocargo that delivers small molecules, as well as a logic sensor for specific signals.[70] Also, Kuzuya and his team have reported an analogous idea but somewhat different effort to a box-shaped 3D origami motif. [71] This approach shows a sophisticated skill, that is, from the initial formation of an open motif, through a stepwise closing process can result in the final box structure.

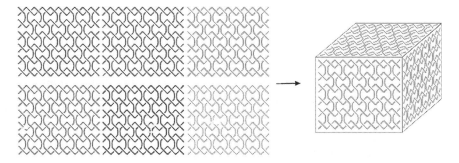

Figure 7. The hexahedral DNA box [70,71]. Six DNA sheets (left) self-assembled into a DNA box [70].

The symmetry properties of DNA cube synthesized by Seeman *et al.* [51] can be conveniently analyzed if the DNA sequences were properly considered. In order to avoid unwanted pairing between DNA strands in the synthesis, the DNA sequences on edges of the DNA cube were designed to have the least symmetry. For example, one of these sequences can be represented as:

$$\frac{\text{CTGCATTCGCCAGCCTGAC}}{\text{GACGTAAGCCGGTCGGACGT}}$$

Obviously, the DNA sequence does not contain any mirror σ and rotation axis C_2. Thus, the DNA cube possesses only C_1 symmetry, i.e., no symmetry. However, the DNA sequence, due to even number of bases involved (20bp), can be redesigned to hold rotational symmetry C_2 by the following way. Reserve the first half sequence and then rotate the helix 180 degrees through the center will generate a DNA palindrome:

$$\frac{\text{CTGCATTCGCCGAATGCAG}}{\text{GACGTAAGCCGGCTTACGTC}}$$

One can easily find that DNA cube consisted of this DNA sequence will conserve O symmetry. Symmetry considerations alone can give us a completely and rigorous answer to the question 'what is possible and what is completely impossible?'. Above results lead us to infer that the DNA octahedra have some features which are regular, and some which are irregular. The symmetry O is very regular whereas the symmetry C_1 is completely irregular. The artificial DNAs are either regular or irregular, whereas the natural DNAs must be irregular. Symmetry means balanced proportions and the high symmetry of molecular structure arising from such balanced proportions. Therefore, artificial DNA with symmetry is easily formed in thermodynamic equilibrium. However, a life system will be open and far from equilibrium, ensuring that molecular symmetry breaking can take place. This explains why the natural DNAs must be irregular and asymmetric.

3.1.3. DNA Octahedron

Octahedron is a good model for DNA nanoconstruction because it provides both regularity and 4-valent connectivity. By now, three complementary methods have been developed to construct DNA octahedron (Shih *et al.*, 2004 [73]; Knudsen *et al.*, 2008 [74], 2010[75]; Mao *et al.*, 2010 [76]). They can be described roughly as 'single-stranded' and 'multi-stranded'.

Shih and his research group have performed an excellent experiment to construct DNA octahedron by folding a 1.7kb long single strand DNA in the presence of five short strands of 40nt.[73] The single long DNA strand first collapse into a branched-tree-like intermediate with the assistance of five short strands, and then fold its branches to form a DNA octahedron (Figure 8a).[73]

The intermediate consists of 5 backbones and 14 branches, each of which is composed of a DNA double-crossover motif (DX)[66] or a half parallel-crossover motif (PX),[77] respectively (Figure 8b). During the annealing process of intermediate, 14 half PXs are paired complementarily to construct seven PXs, as 7 edges of an octahedron, and, associated with 5 DXs, as another 5 edges, to produce the final octahedron.[73] Due to the complex structure of DX and PX motifs, the DNA octahedron can be considered as consisting of two layers.[73] The core layer inside is composed of DNA double helix connected through 4-arm junctions at each vertex, covered with the peripheral layer outside the separated DNA helix on each edge.[73] Thus, each edge of the octahedron consists of a pair of DNA helices, with the one inside containing 40bp and outside 30~35bp, which makes the octahedron much stiffer.[73]

The DNA octahedron contains no catenanes or knots, and can be easily unfolded to a single long DNA strand.[73] Therefore, it can be reproduced by the polymerase chain reaction (PCR), which is crucial for replication of DNA nanostructures.[18]

The construction of DNA octahedron from single-strand-folding strategy wonderfully demonstrates the amazing self-assembly property of DNA in the three-dimensional construction. The main idea of the strategy was improved and demonstrated by Rothemund as a general way to construct DNA polyhedra by folding a single long DNA strand.[78] It is hoped that the strategy will work in laboratory and bring new breakthroughs in DNA nanotechnology.

Recently, Knudsen and colleagues in Denmark constructed DNA octahedron by another approach.[74,75] They designed 8 DNA strands, each containing three subsequences of 18nt linked by 7 unpaired nucleotides.[74] The DNA subsequences are complementary to each other to form DNA helices as edges of the octahedron in the self-assembly process. Because of a larger number of nucleotide linkers involved, the octahedron contains a hole at each vertex (Figure 8c).[74,75] The method is reminiscent of the synthesis of

DNA tetrahedron, and shown to be effective in constructing larger objects, which may serve as DNA cages that suit for drug delivery. These studies are elegant and exciting!

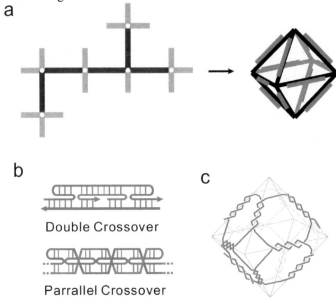

Figure 8. The synthetic strategy and structure of DNA octahedron. (a) DNA octahedron can be formed by folding a branched-tree-like intermediate.[73] Red edges of the intermediate represent DXs and pink edges stand for half PXs. The octahedron contains two layers. The core layer (black) is connected by the 4-armed junctions at vertices. (b) DNA DX (below) and PX (above) can be roughly seen as is composed of parallel DNA double helices. Note that the blue strand in the DX represents short assistant strand. (c) DNA octahedron synthesized by Knudsen et al.[74,75] At each vertex, a hole exists due to the longer unpaired nucleotides (6nt).

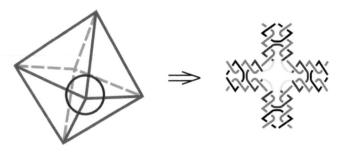

Figure 9. Construction principle of DNA octahedron with '4-point star' motif [76].

Very recently, Mao and coworkers have synthesized DNA octahedra by assembling six well-designed '4-point star' motifs (Figure 9).[76] DNA octahedron with 42bp on each edge was constructed through this method. In addition, length difference of central loops was introduced as a 'experimental reporter' to investigate chiral preference of the self-assembly process.[76] This delicate experiment proposes a new way to surve DNA nanopolyhedra as a model of studying stereochemical process of supermoleular assembly.

The DNA octahedron constructed by Shih *et al.* [73] contains two layers as a core and a peripheral layer. So the DNA sequence on each edge can be represented as:

$$\overline{\text{GCACTTATCCGGACTAGATCCGCTGATCTCGGACGTCGAT}}$$
$$\text{CGTGAATAGCCCTGATCTACGCGACTAGACCCTGCAGCTA}$$

,

$$\overline{\text{CAGGAGCAGGTGCCTCTGATAGCAACCAGGTGAGGA}}$$
$$\text{GTCCTCGTCCACGGAGACTATCGTTGGTCCACTCCT}$$

where the core layer (upper) contains 40bp and the peripheral layer 36bp.[73]

Obviously, the DNA sequence does not contain reflection mirror and rotation axis, and can not be redesigned to be a palindrome due to different lengths of the core and peripheral layer. As a result, the DNA octahedron constructed by Shih *et al.* can only possess the least symmetry C_1.

Another DNA octahedron synthesized by Knudsen's group [74,75] consists of asymmetric sequence such as:

$$\overline{\text{CGATGTCTAAGCTGACCG}}$$
$$\text{GCTACAGATTCGACTGGC}\cdot$$

As a consequence, the DNA octahedron of this sequence is O symmetry. However, due to an even number of bases, it is possible to preserve octahedral symmetry, at least in some extent, by redesigning DNA sequence as follows:

$$\overline{\text{CGATGTCTATAGACATCG}}$$
$$\text{GCTACAGATATCTGTAGC}\cdot$$

It can be proved that DNA octahedron constructed from the above sequence will possess O symmetry.

The edge sequence of DNA octahedron synthesized by Mao *et al.* [76] is represented as:

CCTACGATGGACACGGTAACGCCTAGCAACCTGCCTGGCAAG
GGATGCTACC TGTGCCATTCCGGATCGTTCGACGGACCGTTC

CTTGCCAGGCAGGTTGCTACGCGTTACCGTGTCCATCGTAGG
GAACGGTCCGTCCAACGATCCGCAATGGCACAGGTAGCATCC

Obviously, each edge contains a two-fold rotational axis, which means the DNA octahedron possesses O symmetry.

Symmetry analysis shows that the symmetry of DNA octahedron is transferred from a higher state (O_h) to a lower one (O or C_1). The formation of these lower symmetrical products largely depends on DNA sequences on edges of DNA octahedra. Thus, DNA sequence with C_2 symmetry produces regular DNA octahedron (O), whereas C_1 only gives irregular one (C_1). This is in part because the regular DNA octahedron is formed in quasi-equilibrium process, when the irregular octahedron is produced in thermodynamic process that is far from equilibrium.

3.1.4. DNA Dodecahedron

The synthetic strategy of dodecahedron was proposed by Seeman 10 years ago,[79] however, until recently, DNA dodecahedron was constructed through two different approaches (von Kiedrowski *et al.*, 2008 [80]; Mao *et al.*, 2008 [55]). These syntheses of DNA dodecahedron successfully demonstrated basic strategies of DNA nanoconstruction.

Von Kiedrowski and his fellow researchers have been studying on properties of nonnatural DNA for long time.[81-83] They developed a new branched DNA structure, trisoligonucleotide, which is composed of three DNA single strands covalently linked by an organic molecule, trislinker (Figure 10a). Each trisoligonucleotide, as a novel type of 3-armed DNA junction, contains three unpaired DNA arms that can be joined by complementary DNA arms of others to form larger structures, and thus can be used to construct 3-valent polyhedra (Figure 10). Surprisingly, von Kiedrowski *et al.* have shown that the trisoligonucleotide can replicate itself, as natural DNA, with the existence of complementary DNA strands and organic molecular linkers.

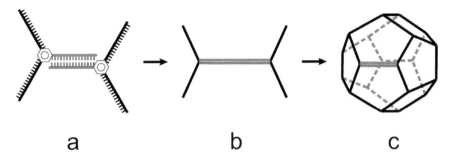

Figure 9. (a) Trisoligonucleotide is composed of three DNA single strands linked to an organic molecule (red). By complementary interactions between ssDNA (a, b), DNA dodecahedron can be formed (c) [80].

In order to construct DNA dodecahedron, 20 trisoligonucleotides were synthesized. Each DNA strand of a trisoligonucleotide contains 15nt and is complementary properly to strands of other trisoligonucleotides to form DNA double helical edges of the dodecahedron.[80] After the annealing process, DNA dodecahedron is produced by the self-assembly of the trisoligonucleotides. Because of the replicable ability of the trisoligonucleotide,[83] it is proposed that the DNA dodecahedron could be reproduced in large amount conveniently, suggesting a possible approach towards the replication of DNA nanostructure.[18, 33]

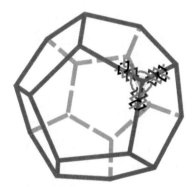

Figure 11. Schematic representation of DNA dodecahedron constructed by the hierarchical self-assembly **process of '3-point star' motifs** [55].

Another approach towards the synthesis of DNA dodecahedron, as a 3-regular **polyhedron, is to assemble 20 '3-point star' motifs, the same tiles** involved in DNA tetrahedron, by hierarchical self-assembly process (Figure 11).[55] By adjusting the unpaired loop to be 3nt and the concentration to be

50nM, Mao and colleagues successfully synthesized DNA dodecahedra in the annealing process with 76% yield.[55] The DNA dodecahedron here contains parallel DNA double helices of 42bp, 4nm on each edge, which is consistent with the observation in cryo-EM experiment.[55] This is still an exciting challenging, and there is a window for new ideas and new theories interested in this important field.

The DNA sequence of DNA dodecahedron synthesized by von Kiedrowski *et al.*[80] can be written as:

$$\frac{\text{CCTGTCTTGAACGAG}}{\text{GGACAGAACTTGCTC}} \cdot$$

It does not contain any reflection mirror and rotation axis, and can not be redesigned because of 15 base pairs involved. As a result, DNA dodecahedron synthesized with this kind of DNA sequence possesses only C_1 symmetry. However, the DNA dodecahedron constructed with '3-point star' motif contains each edge with DNA sequence as:

$$\frac{\text{CCTACGATGGACACGGTAACGCCTAGCAACCTGCCTGGCAAG}}{\text{GGATGCTACCTGTGCCATTCCGGATCGTTCGACGGACCGTTC}} \cdot$$

$$\frac{\text{CTTGCCAGGCAGGTTGCTACGCGTTACCGTGTCCATCGTAGG}}{\text{GAACGGTCCGTCCAACGATCCGCAATGGCACAGGTAGCATCC}}$$

Apparently, a two-fold rotational axis exists at the center of the sequence. And thus, we can conclude that DNA dodecahedron made by Mao *et al.*[55] has *I* symmetry.

Consideration of the point symmetry groups has led to the discovery of a new way to understand symmetry and asymmetry of nanopolyhedra. The point symmetry group of DNA dodecahedra belongs to *I* or C_1 group, indicating the loss of either reflection mirror or rotational axis. The process $I \rightarrow C_1$ is referred to as molecular symmetry breaking,[68] which means a system goes from a symmetric state to an asymmetric one. Molecular symmetry breaking may be a basis of characterizing the complexity and variety of the medically and biologically most interesting DNAs.

3.1.5. DNA Icosahedron

Icosahedron is the most complex structure in Platonic polyhedra, and, due to its 5-valent vertex, beyond the binding abilities of common chemical bond, is a formidable challenge for chemical synthesis. However, with the help of DNA, three groups have constructed icosahedron at molecular scale (Mao *et al.*, 2008 [84]; Shih *et al.*, 2009 [85]; Krishnan *et al.*, 2009 [86]), suggesting a laudable approach towards mimicking nature.

It is believed before that, in order to construct complex polyhedron, each motif must have enough rigidity so that the geometric object could be built like tinker-toys.[84] However, Mao's group designed a more flexible tile, '5-point star' with unpaired loop of 5nt, and utilized the tiles to perform the amazing synthesis (Figure 12).[84] Surprisingly, DNA icosahedron was successfully integrated, and after AFM test, the icosahedron was proved to possess good rigidity, which demonstrates appropriate flexibility of DNA motifs is helpful in the DNA nanoconstruction of complex structures.[84]

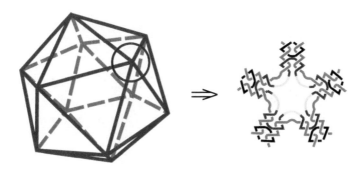

Figure 12. Synthetic principle of DNA icosahedron [84].

More recently, Shih's group have extended two-dimensional scaffold DNA origami to build complex three-dimensional structures.[85] They have constructed a DNA icosahedron with three 'double-triangule' intermediates in a two-step hierarchical self-assembly process (Figure 13).[85] Besides, a series of three-dimensional nanostructures have been also created by the same method, which indicates an effective approach towards systematic three-dimensional DNA nanoconstrucion. These important successes of DNA polyhedra lead to new goals for future research in chemical synthesis, but we have only explored a minuscule fraction of this new domain!

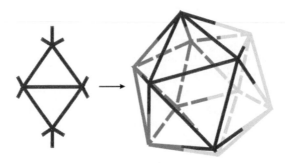

Figure 13. DNA icosahedron constructed from three 'double-triangle' structures (left) [85].

The DNA icosahedron synthesized by Mao *et al.* [84] contains 12 identical '5-point star' motifs and identical DNA sequence on each edge as:

CCTACGATGGACACGGTAACGCCTAGCAACCTGCCTGGCAAG
GGATGCTACCTGTGCCATTCCGGATCGTTCGACGGACCGTTC

CTTGCCAGGCAGGTTGCTACGCGTTACCGTGTCCATCGTAGG
GAACGGTCCGTCCAACGATCCGCAATGGCACAGGTAGCATCC

Because the sequence contains a C_2 axis, it can be proved that the DNA icosahedron has the point group I. The most highly symmetrical presentation has led to the discovery of a new way to consider molecular design of the novel nanopolyhedra.

In general case, mathematical polyhedra are highly symmetric, and this is why they stand for pure beauties. DNA polyhedra, due to the mechanism of molecular symmetry breaking, are usually in a lower symmetric state, or even completely asymmetric. DNA icosahedron analyzed here belongs to I group, because it contains no reflection mirrors. This I symmetry group tells us that molecular model of DNA nanopolyhedra always lacks a plane of symmetry, and therefore is said to possess chirality or handedness in a chemical word.

3.2. ARCHIMEDEAN SOLIDS

Archimedean polyhedron, different from Platonic polyhedron, is semi-regular in that each face of the polyhedron is regular but several kinds of faces exist (Figure 14). There are 13 Archimedean solids. However, until now, only two of them, truncated octahedron and truncated icosahedron, were successfully synthesized with DNA.[2] The truncated octahedron and truncated icosahedron possesses O_h and I_h symmetry respectively, and the symmetry of corresponding DNA polyhedra are, of course, decided by the DNA sequences involved.

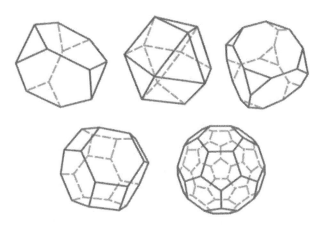

Figure 14. Some of the Archimedean solids. They are, in successive, truncated tetrahedron, truncated octahedron, truncated cube, truncated dodecahedron, and truncated icosahedron.

3.2.1. DNA Truncated Octahedron

The truncated octahedron is derived from octahedron by truncating each vertex, which is composed of eight triangles and six hexagons (Figure 15a).

Although the object contains only 3-valent vertices, however, in order to obtain larger structures in 3-space, Seeman's group [52] utilized 4-armed DNA junctions in the construction, leaving an extra arm at each vertex. Six squares of the truncated octahedron were synthesized first to obtain an intermediate, which can be used to construct the final structure (Figure 15b).[52] If the extra arms were properly ligated, it may produce a three-dimensional lattice structure with the truncated octahedron as repeating units.[52] And with the help of the extra arms, it is believed that the DNA truncated octahedron might prefer a configuration with the extra arms face outside, indicating good stereochemical control (Figure 15c).[52] The final DNA truncated octahedron contains 20bp on each edge, i.e. 6.8nm, and consists of 14 rings, each of ~1000nt.[52] This is a monumental achievement in the history of the DNA nanopolyhedra world!

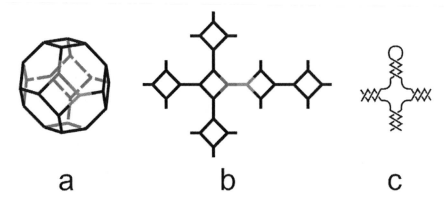

Figure 15. Schematic illustrations of DNA truncated octahedron (a), intermediate with six squares (b) and DNA junctions used in the synthesis (c) [52].

The DNA sequence of DNA truncated octahedron can be written as:

GCAGAGTGGTTCTCACTAGT
CGTCTCACCAAGAGTGATCA

Because of lacking reflection mirror and rotation axis, the point symmetry group of DNA truncated octahedron degenerates from O_h to C_1. However, if reconstructed the DNA truncated octahedron with the sequence:

GCAGAGTGGTACCACTCTGC
CGTCTCACCATGGTGAGACG

an O symmetry group will be reserved at least. Such symmetry highlights an order and coherence in the working of nanopolyhedra.

3.2.2. DNA Truncated Icosahedron

The truncated icosahedron, which contains 32 faces and 60 vertices, is a fascinating structure that has arisen many chemical interests. Such a structure is well-known by soccer ball and molecular buckminsterfullerene (buckyball, or fullerene C_{60}).[38] Synthesizing DNA buckyball is a particular challenge that could have very important results for chemists.

Mao and colleagues have constructed the DNA buckyball,[55] or DNA truncated icosahedron, with the help of the hierarchical self-assembly strategy. They have employed sixty '3-point star' motifs in the synthesis, as vertices of the truncated icosahedron (Figure 16). By controlling the concentration of motifs at 500nM and the unpaired loop of 3nt, the DNA truncated icosahedra were obtained with a yield of 69%.[55] The structure of the products was examined with the AFM analysis and cryo-EM technique. The possibility of molecular realization of larger geometric polyhedra may provide basis for drug delivery and nanoreactors. This is an especially exciting development for chemistry, and this discovery would mark a beginning, not an end. The most creative act in chemistry is the design and creation of new nanopolyhedra. The challenge is picking the right targets, as well as figuring out how to make them.

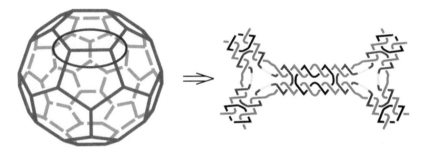

Figure 16. DNA truncated icosahedron (left) is built by the linkages of '3-point star' motifs (right) [55].

The DNA buckyball possesses I symmetry. This can be seen by analyzing its sequence structure, which can be represented as:

CCTACGATGGACACGGTAACGCCTAGCAACCTGCCTGGCAAG
GGATGCTACCTGTGCCATTCCGGATCGTTCGACGGACCGTTC
CTTGCCAGGCAGGTTGCTACGCGTTACCGTGTCCATCGTAGG
GAACGGTCCGTCCAACGATCCGCAATGGCACAGGTAGCATCC

Obviously, the sequence contains a C_2 axis at its center. So, the symmetry analysis of DNA truncated icosahedron is valuable according to the discussion in Section 3.1.

3.3. MORE COMPLICATED POLYHEDRA

3.3.1. DNA Prisms and Bipyramid

The chemical synthesis of DNA prisms and bipyramid was one of the biggest challenges in DNA nanotechnology due to lower point symmetry group, i.e. D_{nd} group (Figure 17).[2] Sleiman's group and Turberfield's group have been working on this topic, and, both using their strategies, synthesized a series of DNA prisms and bipyramid for a demonstration (Sleiman *et al.*, 2007 [87]; Turberfield *et al.*, 2007 [88]).

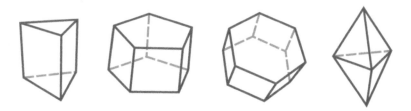

Figure 17. Several prisms and bipyramid. From left to right, they are triangular prism, pentagonal prism, hexagonal prism and bipyramid.

Sleiman and colleagues have developed a systematic strategy to construct a library of prisms.[87] They have constructed a few DNA polygons that contain several DNA strands as edges linked by organic molecules at vertices, as molecular modules for further construction.[87] With help of several DNA single-strands as linkers, these polygonal modules can be combined to produce a series of prisms (Figure 18). Furthermore, the DNA polygons with organic molecules involved were shown to be more rigid than branched DNA junctions, which made DNA prisms more stable.[89, 90]

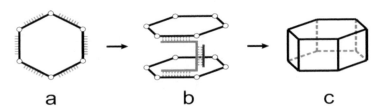

a   b   c

Figure 18. DNA polygon, hexagons for example here, is consisted of several ssDNAs connected through organic molecules (small ball) (a). DNA prisms (c) can be generated by joining polygonal modules with long strand DNA as linker (b, green) and short DNA as stiffer (b, red) [87].

They have utilized DNA strands of 10nt and certain number of organic molecules to synthesize four structure modules, triangles, squares, pentagons and hexagons.[87] And with the assistant of DNA linker strands of 30nt and 10nt, a library of DNA prisms have been constructed, including DNA triangular prism, cube, pentagonal and hexagonal prism, biprisms and heteroprisms, and structurally swichable prism.[87] The geometry parameters of these objects are summarized in Table 2. It is notable that, in principle, any structures that can be retrosynthetically broke down into these DNA modules can be reconstructed, which provides a systematic synthetic approach to DNA nanoconstruction.[87]

Table 2. Edge parameters of DNA prisms

DNA prisms	Geometer parameters
Triangular, quadrangular, pentagonal, hexagonal prism	face edge: 10bp side edge: 10bp
Heteroprism and biprism[*]	face edge: 10bp side edge: 20bp
Edge switchable prism	face edge: 10bp side edge: (10,14,20)bp[**]

* Heteroprism here is composed of a triangular face and a hexagonal face, while biprism is the combination of two heteroprisms, by gluing the hexagonal faces. ** (10, 14, 20)bp means the edge length of the switchable prism is varied within 10, 14, or 20bp.[87]

Another polyhedron with rotation symmetry, bipyramid, is a common model in chemistry, serving as a geometric model for molecular orbital structure. Although the bipyramid contains only nine edges and five vertices, it is still difficult to construct such a structure because of its irregular vertex valences, two of which are 3-valent and the other three are 4. However, Turberfield's work [88] have recently constructed DNA bipyramid by the self-assembly of several DNA strands. They designed six single strands, each consisting of three subsequences of 20nt joined by one unpaired nucleotide (Figure 19).[88] In the annealing process, six strands combined each other through the complementarity of DNA subsequences, to form DNA bipyramid. The bipyramid contains 20bp on each edge and six nicks on six of its edges.[88]

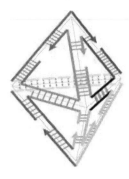

Figure 19. DNA bipyramid is consisted of six ssDNAs (different colors) with each running around a triangular face. Six of the edges contain a nick [88].

The DNA sequences of DNA prisms and DNA bipyramid can be represented as:

$$\frac{\text{CCGATTTGTG}}{\text{GGCTAAACAC}}$$

and

$$\frac{\text{CGAACATTCCTAAGTCTGAA}}{\text{GCTTGTAAGGATTCAGACTT}},$$

respectively. Because they both have the least symmetry, the DNA prisms and bipyramid will thus possess only C_1 symmetry or no symmetry. However, the replacement of these sequences with

$$\frac{\text{CCGATATCGG}}{\text{GGCTATAGCC}}$$

and

$$\frac{\text{CGAACATTCCGGAATGTTCG}}{\text{GCTTGTAAGGCCTTACAAGC}}$$

will reserve D_{nd} and D_3 symmetry for prisms and bipyramid, respectively. Since the symmetry has provided a powerful and insightful guidance, chemists usually rely on such an approach to help themselves understand molecular structures.

3.3.2. Goldberg Polyhedra

Goldberg polyhedra are a class of complex polyhedra, which can be generated and constructed in an infinite way (Figure 20). They are composed of pentagons and hexagons only, and the number of its faces is described by following formulas:[37]

$$F_5 = 12 \, ;$$
$$F_6 = 10 \times (h^2 + hk + k^2 - 1) \, ,$$

where F_5 and F_6 represent the number of pentagons and hexagons, and h, k are integers.

The construction of a series of Goldberg polyhedra in a systematic and efficient way is a charming but formidable challenge in chemistry. Fortunately, the two smallest Goldberg polyhedra, i.e. dodecahedron (h=1, k=0; Figure 11) and truncated icosahedron (h=1, k=1; Figure 16) have been constructed (von Kiedrowski et $al.$, 2008 [80]; Mao et $al.$, 2008 [55]). It is an interesting phenomenon that the geometry of Goldberg polyhedra can be used to describe and classify the most number of spherical viral capsid structure.[11, 40] As a example, the virus HK97 of particular scientific interests is a 72-hedron (h=2, k=1).[15, 16] Therefore, chemical synthesis with Goldberg polyhedra as a structural framework is considered to be a natural and infinite way towards mimicking nature, and may lead to our further understanding of viral capsids. Progress is real, but the goal line is still some distance down the field.

Figure 20. Some examples of Goldberg polyhedra. They are composed of 12 pentagons and certain numbers of hexagons. From left to right are 12-hedron, 32-hedron, 72-hedron, and 92-hedron separately.

4. POLYHEDRAL LINKS –
NOVEL STRUCTURES
FROM DNA POLYHEDRA

DNA nanopolyhedra have extended our idea of what is possible in the chemical and biological world, since no such structures exist in nature. The construction of polyhedral structures with DNA improves the development of synthetic chemistry, and meanwhile, produces some complicated molecules with novel topological and geometrical structures, such as the DNA tetrahedron [53-55], DNA cube [51], DNA octahedron [73-75], DNA dodecahedron [55, 80], DNA icosahedron [84-86], and the DNA buckyball [55], as well as the tetrahedron DNA cage [56] and the cube DNA box [70,71], etc.... These are some monumental feats and achievements! A challenge that is just now being addressed concerns how to ascertain and comprehend some of the mysterious characteristics of the DNA polyhedral folding.

Studies with DNA nanopolyhedra indicate that ordinary geometry is replaced by something known as nanopolyhedral geometry and topology. In this geometrical framework, the conventional notions of space and of distance between points melt away, leaving us in a vastly different mathematical apparatus and conceptual innovations. It is always better to know exactly that a polyhedron is a solid of the three-dimensional space limited by a finite number of the faces, the edges and the vertices. More curiously, a DNA nanopolyhedron is an interlocked and interlinked structure with the polyhedral skeleton: the edges are assembled with 2-helix and 4-helix, and so on; the vertices and the faces are filled with 'holes' that are small, and the others large. It is surprising to discover that the small 'holes' are the molecular skeletons, whereas the large 'holes' are a network of tunnels as if some 'creatures' travel through them.[34, 91, 96] Within this new framework, the marriage of the large and the small 'holes' will result in a stunning revision of our understanding of the DNA three-dimensional shapes, aesthetically pleasing sculptures, and functional devices and materials. The new elements, helices and holes, have changed the properties of original polyhedra in a number of ways. Therefore, DNA nanopolyhedra have no faces, no edges, and no vertices. Because these feature of DNA nanopolyhedra require that we drastically change our understanding of new architectures. These interesting objects challenge the mathematical theory of polyhedra and indicate an undiscovered geometry and topology. There are many important questions waiting to be answered, and further explorations are needed! The progress will require the creation of better tools and better theories.

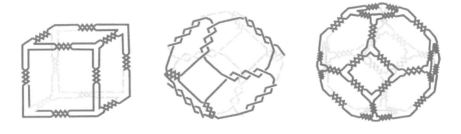

Figure 21. Schematic illustrations of [6]-catenanes (DNA cube), [8]-catenanes (DNA octahedron) and [14]-catenanes (DNA truncated octahedron).

The DNA nanopolyhedra world is so vast and complex that it is now necessary to clarify the definitions to describe topologically interlinked and interlocked cases (Figure 21). The best way to gain a good understanding of the different types of DNA nanopolyhedral architectures is to use a set of models. Since 2005, Qiu's group has proposed and constructed a novel topological and geometrical structure, i.e. polyhedral links, to model the molecular structure of DNA polyhedra, and, with the help of graph theory and knot theory, characterized and analyzed the mathematical properties of these polyhedral links.[34] Some interesting properties, such as chirality and duality, have been uncovered. As a result, these beautiful architectures are now updating our knowledge of the geometry of polyhedra, and improving pure mathematical theory, such as graph theory and knot theory.[92-95] Meanwhile, the systematic knowledge of polyhedral links may also provide new insights into biomolecular structures, such as viral capsids and DNA polyhedra.[15, 16, 21-25]   The architecture of the polyhedra links builds an inexhaustible spring of inspiration for geometry thinking and to illustrate the research in topology. Although there is much to learn, the idea is simple but brilliant, as many excellent academic ideas are.

4.1. PLATONIC POLYHEDRAL LINKS

Platonic solids are the simplest ones in the polyhedral world. However, they present some of the basic concepts of polyhedra, such as vertex degree and duality. Qiu's group has developed two basic transformations, 'n-branched curves and k-twisted line covering' and 'n-crossover and k-twisted line covering', to systematically generate and construct a series of polyhedral links based on the geometry of Platonic polyhedra.[34, 91, 96] Furthermore, interesting properties such as knot invariant and dual transformation are investigated and explored.[96-98]

It is now clear that polyhedral link is an interlocked cage with holes or tunnels, whose boundaries, of course, are the double- or multi-helix that has the even or odd number of half-twists. More curiously, the vertex area with holes of the polyhedral link is a novel position of topology which controls molecular shape or size.[34,91,96]

4.1.1. Type I Platonic Polyhedral Links and Knot Invariants

The first type of Platonic polyhedral links was generated on the Platonic polyhedra by the method of 'n-branched curves and k-twisted line covering'. The basic geometric elements that composed of Platonic polyhedra, vertices, edges and faces, were replaced by novel complex motifs, 'n-branched curves', 'k-twisted line' and holes that connect the inside and outside of the polyhedra,[91,96] respectively. After the transformation, the Type I Platonic polyhedral links were obtained (Figure 22).[96]

The vertex degree of the first type of Platonic polyhedral links is varied only among 3-, 4- and 5-valent. However, the twist number on edge motif 'k-twisted line' can be changed infinitely in both directions, which will produce a series of 'topological isomers' (Figure 23).[91,96] To classify all these possible isomers need the structural characterization by knot invariants. Knot invariant is a mathematical quantity that can depict the characters of topological isomers, such as crossing number, writhe number, linking number, and HOMFLY polynomial.[92-95, 99-104] It can be used to, at least in principle, identify tiny differences between similar structures, and therefore, **distinguish and classify the 'topological isomers'. Qiu and co**-workers have computed these knot invariants of the type I Platonic polyhedral links, which may be helpful for further classification and characterization.[96]

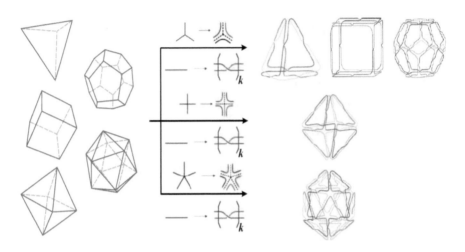

Figure 22. The first type of Platonic polyhedral links **are obtained by using** '3-branched curves and k-twisted line covering', '4-branched curves and k-twisted **line covering'**, **and** '5-branched curves and k-twisted **line covering' according to the corresponding** vertex degree of Platonic polyhedra.[34,91,96] Here, polyhedral links are presented with k=1.

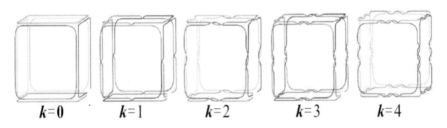

$k=0$ $k=1$ $k=2$ $k=3$ $k=4$

Figure 23. Representations of hexahedral links in the case of k=0, 1, 2, 3, and 4. Platonic polyhedral links with different twist number k result in a series of different 'topological isomers' [91,96].

4.1.2. Type II Platonic Polyhedral Links
and Dual Transformation

In the second type of Platonic polyhedral links, edges and vertices of polyhedra are replaced by '*n*-crossover' and '*k*-twisted line', respectively (Figure 24b). Because of different motifs used in generation, the topological structure of the second type of polyhedral links is completely different from the first type. And interestingly, five type II Platonic polyhedral links can be converted from each other by dual transformations (Figure 24a, b).[97-98]

In geometry, duality means the vertices and faces can be exchanged between a pair of polyhedra. So, in the Platonic polyhedra, the octahedron and the cube, the dodecahedron and the icosahedron, the tetrahedron and itself, are considered to be dual polyhedra respectively (Figure 24a).[2] Surprisingly, dual relationships also exist in the Platonic polyhedral links, and can be classified as two types, i.e. trivial and nontrivial.[97-98] Dual transformation is said to be trivial if the geometric motifs of dual polyhedral links remain unchanged, otherwise, nontrivial. Therefore, the dual transformation between the tetrahedral links and itself is trivial. And the others belong to the realm of nontrivial, for the different construction methods, i.e. '4-crossover and 2-twisted line covering', '5-crossover and 2-twisted line covering' and '3-crossover and 2-twisted line covering', are connected through the dual transformations (Figure 24b).[97-98]

Based on these interesting results, Qiu's group has generalized the dual transformations of polyhedral links.[98] In graph theory, a three-dimensional polyhedron can be represented by a two-dimensional graph, Schlegel diagram, and furthermore, a pair of dual polyhedra can be connected through medial graphs on Schlegel diagrams.[101-102] Medial graphs, according to mathematical graph theory, have such properties that each vertex in the graph is 4-valent and the faces of the graph can be painted with two different colors. This is somewhat like a chessboard that contains two colors of squares and has four directions on each vertex without respect to the outmost lines. In the case of polyhedra, the medial graphs can be obtained by connecting medial points on edges if two edges are neighboured through a vertex. And it can be proved by mathematical techniques that the medial graphs of a pair of dual polyhedra are the same, and *vice versa*.[102]

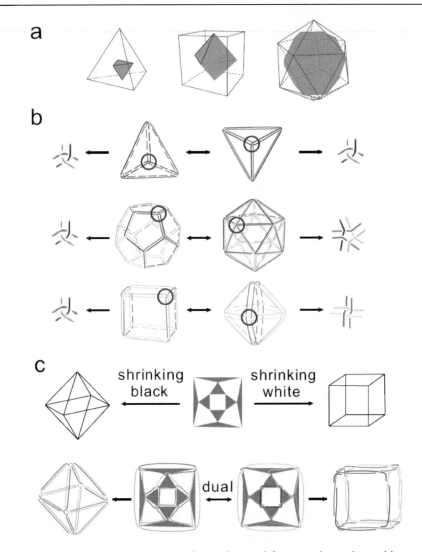

Figure 24. (a) Dual polyhedra means the vertices and faces can be exchanged between a pair of polyhedra. (b) Dual Platonic polyhedral links can be classified as trivial (above) and nontrivial (medium and below), with the difference that the former does not change the geometric motifs that composed of polyhedral links while nontrivial not. (c) Construction principle of dual polyhedral links. A pair of dual polyhedra, for example cube and octahedron, can be connected by the medial graph of their Schlegel diagram (above). Fill the opposite faces of the medial graph with two colors, say black and white. And covering the 4-valent vertex of the graph with '2-twisted line' in the manner either across the white (below, left) or black area (below, right) will produce two different kinds of medial graph links. Shrinking the white or black area then gives hexahedral or octahedral links respectively [97].

Covering each vertex of the medial graph of polyhedra with 'k-twisted line' motifs, and connecting the ends of adjoined motifs will produce catenaned structures, medial graph links (Figure 24c). It is notable that there are two choices of the arrangement of 'k-twisted line', either crossing through the white or black faces, as well as two types of medial graph links. And these two types of links can be topologically transformed into a pair of dual polyhedral links (Figure 24c). The dual polyhedral links constructed by the method can be classified into two categories, which are O-dual if the twist number k is odd and E-dual otherwise.[98]

Although the knowledge of dual polyhedral links is still limited now, it is believed that duality, one of the most profound concepts in nature, will bring some new ideas in the study of polyhedral links, such as classification and topological transformation.

4.2. TRUNCATED PLATONIC POLYHEDRAL LINKS, ARCHIMEDEAN POLYHEDRAL LINKS AND CHIRALITY

Archimedean polyhedra and truncated Platonic polyhedra are two classes of 3-regular polyhedra, which can be generated by truncating vertices of Platonic polyhedra once or several times respectively (Figure 25a).[1, 2] Qiu's group has used the method of '3-crossover and k-twisted line covering' to construct a series of polyhedral links (Figure 25b), which can be characterized by some mathematical recursive formulas.[91]

All these polyhedral links are showed to be chiral by symmetry analysis. A polyhedron is said to be chiral if it cannot be superimposed onto its mirror image. Because of the rigidity of polyhedra, it is easy to decide whether a polyhedron is chiral or not, by the analysis of its improper rotation symmetry. For a catenaned structure with sufficient flexibility like rubber, however, the criterion can no longer insist due to the definition of rotation axis in topological sense. Some of the catenanes seemed lacking of improper rotations could be deformed into its 'mirror image' by stretching and shrinking, just like a transformation between left and right hand as a topological rubber glove (Figure 26a).[68] Therefore, deciding whether topologically catenaned structures, say polyhedral links, possessing chirality is a more difficult task.[68, 103, 104]

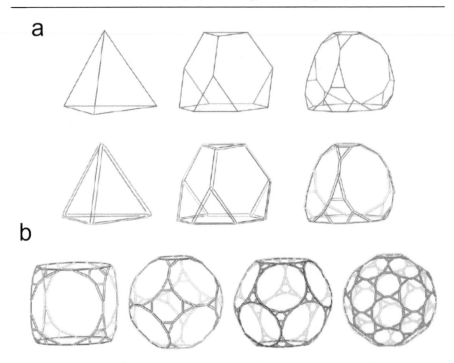

Figure 25. (a) Truncated tetrahedra generated by a series of truncating operations on tetrahedron (above), and their corresponding polyhedral links. (b) Polyhedral links obtained by truncating cube, octahedron, dodecahedron and icosahedron twice, and then with '3-crossover and double twisted line covering'.[91]

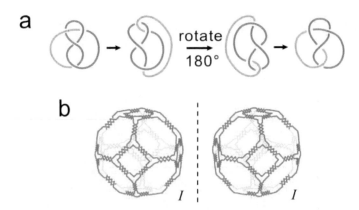

Figure 26. (a) Under the topological transformations, the 'figure eight' knot can be transformed into its 'mirror image'. (b) truncated octahedral links exist as two mirror images.

In fact, mathematicians have been working for years to develop techniques to probe the topological chirality of molecular catenanes and graphs. A number of techniques, such as knot polynomial calculation, point symmetry group analysis of Seifert construction, 2-fold branched covering and Möbius ladder analysis, are useful in simple knots with a few crossovers.[68, 105-114] However, it is not convenient to apply these techniques in determining whether a polyhedral links is chiral.

Qiu and his team have proposed a new technique in chriality determination by analyzing point symmetry group of polyhedral links. It is believed that point group of polyhedral links and corresponding polyhedra are the same except for the mirror reflection elements. So, the symmetry group of a polyhedral link is usually T, O or I. Thus, it can be concluded empirically that polyhedral links are chiral in general cases (Figure 26b).[34, 91] Recent studies on polynomials of some of the polyhedral links give the same results.[115] This empirical method, if proved mathematically, will be convenient and helpful for the characterization of molecular symmetry breaking of DNA polyhedra.[68]

4.3. GOLDBERG POLYHEDRAL LINKS

Novel geometric objects such as Platonic polyhedral links and Archimedean polyhedral links provide a foundation for the characterization and analysis of DNA polyhedra synthesized in laboratory. Meanwhile, it opens a door for the realm of polyhedral links. In order to explore general principles and mechanisms of these fantastic structures, Qiu *et al.* have constructed a great number of polyhedral links based on the geometry of Goldberg polyhedra, which may be useful to our understanding of biomacromolecules, such as viral capsids.[15, 16, 34]

4.3.1. Goldberg Polyhedral Links

Goldberg polyhedra are complex polyhedra and thus have infinite numbers of different structures.[37] However, there exist two types that are relatively simple, which can be described by the following recursive formulas:[34]

Type I: $F_{n+1} = F_n + 10(2n+1)$;

Type II: $F_{n+1} = F_n + 20n$,

where F_n represents the faces of Goldberg polyhedra.

Based on the geometry of the two types of Goldberg polyhedra and the method of '3-crossover and k-twisted line covering', Qiu's group has constructed two types of Goldberg polyhedral links. Structural analysis shows that they are interlocked catenanes of certain numbers of pentagonal and hexagonal rings. The numbers of component rings satisfy the following relations (Figure 27):[34]

Type I: $R_{n+1} = R_n + 10(2n+1)$;

Type II: $R_{n+1} = R_n + 20n$,

where R_n is the number of interlocked rings.

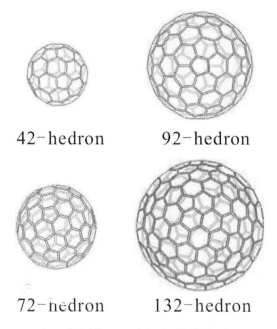

42-hedron   92-hedron

72-hedron   132-hedron

Figure 27. Some examples of Goldberg polyhedra.[34] The lower row represents type II Goldberg polyhedral links, which contain a 72-hedron as a mathematical model for the molecular topological structure of the capsid protein of virus HK97.

Symmetry analysis indicates that the two types of Goldberg polyhedral links are all chiral, which is the property different from Goldberg polyhedra. Amazingly, the structure of Goldberg polyhedral links with $n=2$ in the second type is coincident with the topological architecture of capsid protein of virus HK97, consisting of 12 pentagonal and 60 hexagonal rings (Figure 27).[15, 16] This interesting discovery indicates some common mechanisms of molecular structures. Further investigations will bring additional insights into the structures of biomacromolecules.

4.3.2. Extended Goldberg Polyhedra and Polyhedral Links

Base on the first and second type of Goldberg polyhedra, Qiu *et al.* have used two operations, namely 'spherical rotating' and 'spherical stretching', to construct Rotate-Extended Goldberg Polyhedra (REGP) and Stretch-Extended Goldberg Polyhedra (SEGP), respectively (Figure 28).[116] Except for the pentagons and hexagons contained in the original Goldberg polyhedra, the REGPs are also composed of certain numbers of triangles, whereas the SEGPs consist of triangles and squares. These two types of extended Goldberg polyhedra can be characterized by the following recursive relations:[116]

Type I:

REGP: $F_n = 12 + 10(n^2 + 2n) + 20(n+1)^2$;

SEGP: $F_n = 12 + 10(n^2 + 2n) + 50(n+1)^2$;

Type II:

REGP: $F_n = 12 + 10(n^2 + n) + 20(n^2 + n + 1)$;

SEGP: $F_n = 12 + 10(n^2 + n) + 50(n^2 + n + 1)$,

where F_n represents the faces of extended Goldberg polyhedra.

The vertex valences of all the two types of extended Goldberg polyhedra are 4, which can be covered with 'k-twisted line' motifs to produce two classes of extended Goldberg polyhedral links, i.e. Rotate-Extended Goldberg Polyhedral Links (REGPL) and Stretch-Extended Goldberg Polyhedral links (SEGPL) (Figure 28).[117, 118] Different from Goldberg polyhedral links, the number of the interlocked rings depends on the twist number k of the motifs.

In the case that k is even, the each component ring runs along a face in the extended Goldberg polyhedron. And thus, the number of rings can be calculated by the following deductions:[117, 118]

Type I:

REGPL: $R_n = 12 + 10(n^2 + 2n) + 20(n+1)^2$;

SEGPL: $R_n = 12 + 10(n^2 + 2n) + 50(n+1)^2$;

Type II:

REGPL: $R_n = 12 + 10(n^2 + n) + 20(n^2 + n + 1)$;

SEGPL: $R_n = 12 + 10(n^2 + n) + 50(n^2 + n + 1)$,

where R_n represents the component rings of extended Goldberg polyhedral links.

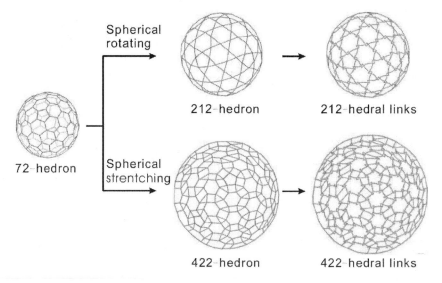

Figure 28. By applying the 'spherical rotating' and 'spherical stretching' operations on Goldberg polyhedra, Rotate-Extended Goldberg Polyhedra (REGP) and Stretch-Extended Goldberg Polyhedra (SEGP) are obtained.[117] Then, by the following 'k-twisted line covering', Rotate-Extended Goldberg Polyhedral Links (REGPL) and Stretch-Extended Goldberg Polyhedral links will be generated respectively.[118] Here, k=2, for examples.

In the case of an odd k, it can be only ascertained that the component rings are less than that when k is even. However, to calculate the number of rings in analytic manner is quite difficult for the reason that each ring will encompass through certain number of faces.[119-122] Qiu *et al.* have proposed an algorithm to compute the component rings in some special cases.[118] Meanwhile, Twarock *et al.* are seeking a different mathematical tool, topological graph theory, to solve such a problem. [123] With the help of a computer, they have established relationships between component numbers and some other topological invariants and then give an interesting result. For a dodecahedral and an icosidodecahedral link (32-hedral link), the least numbers of rings are both two.[123-125]

The computation and exploration of the number of component rings is not merely a mathematical issue, but can also work as theoretical blueprints in the design of experiments. DNA polyhedra with minimal number of strands can be easily replicated by PCR, which is meaningful in DNA nanotechnology and even crucial to some RNA virus genome packing. [18, 126- 132]

Chapter 5

5. CONCLUSION

The study of polyhedra is a very old subject. However, chemists have refreshed this issue in laboratory while employing smart DNA as a nanoconstruction material.[1, 2, 21-25] DNA cube synthesized by Seeman et al. [51] has greatly inspired chemists' imagination. In the past two decades, they have utilized DNA to construct a great number of polyhedra from a simple cube to a more complex buckyball. These novel structures of DNA polyhedra have improved our knowledge on the basic forms of molecular structures, bringing insightful ideas to understand mechanisms of biomacromolecules, such as viral capsids. The future interest in these species needs urgent investigation, because of not only their application in nanotechnology, but also their intriguing topologies, which remind us of the reflections on the new theories of polyhedra.

Polyhedral links, the interlinked and interlocked architectures, have extended our ideas of what the potential shape of polyhedral molecules is. The review that presents the theoretical study of polyhedral links involves the following five major endeavors: (1) the exploration of a systematic mathematical transformation to construct polyhedral links on any given polyhedra; (2) the elucidation of duality in the new form of polyhedra, i.e. polyhedral links; (3) the detection of the chirality of polyhedral links and their applications in the synthesis and characterization of new forms of DNA and protein molecules; (4) the usage of topology and graph theory to understand the symmetry and asymmetry of polyhedral links; and (5) the elucidation and computation of the number of component rings with the help of topological graph theory.

However, the story has just begun. There is still a gap between relatively simple theoretical systems and the complicated varieties of DNA supramolecular polyhedra, such as DNA buckyball. Some problems of general interests have not been solved and even proposed yet. For instances, how to generate more complex polyhedra on the simple polyhedra (e.g. Platonic solids) and what the general principle of the geometry and topology of polyhedral links is.[34, 91, 96-98, 115-118, 133-136] Such problems, though they are strange enough, still lead us to a higher level of the understanding to the characteristics of polyhedral molecules (e.g. DNA polyhedra and viral capsids), such as intramolecular symmetry breaking,[68] providing available opportunities for the development of a mathematical theory of new geometry.

In conclusion, the interactions between chemical and mathematical concerns on DNA polyhedra benefit and promote each other well. It is our belief that further study on these beautiful molecules will serve an arena for the interdisciplinary improvement between chemistry and mathematics. In fact, the scope for new research in mathematical chemistry is so broad that full and cooperative endeavors from mathematics [137-138] and chemistry are warranted and required. Mathematical chemistry, or biomathematics, must provide the basic knowledge for the next cycle of new discovery and development. How important such study will be remains to be seen! However, we have explored only a minuscule fraction of this new domain.

ACKNOWLEDGEMENTS

This work was supported by Grants from the National Natural Science Foundation of China (No. 20973085 and No.10831001) and Specialized Research Fund for the Doctoral Program of Higher Education of China (No. 20090211110006).

REFERENCES

[1]   Coxeter, H. M. S. (1973). *Regular Polytopes*. Dover: Dover Publications.

[2]   Cromwell, P. R. (1999). *Polyhedra: "One of the Most Charming Chapters of Geometry"*. Cambridge: Cambridge University Press.

[3]   Hargittai, I. & Hargittai, M. (1995). *Symmetry Through the Eyes of a Chemist*. New York: Plenum Press.

[4]   Maier, G., Pfriem, S., Schäfer, U. & Matusch, R. (1978). Tetra-tert-butyltetrahedrane. *Angew. Chem., Int. Ed.*, 17, 520-521.

[5]   Eaton, P. E. & Cole, T. W. (1964). The cubane system. *J. Am. Chem. Soc.*, 86, 962-964.

[6]   Eaton, P. E. & Cole, T. W. (1964). Cubane. *J. Am. Chem. Soc.*, 86, 3157-3158.

[7]   Paquette, L. A., Balogh, D. W., Usha, R., Kountz, D. & Christoph, G. G. (1981). Crystal and molecular structure of a pentagonal dodecahedrane. *Science*, 211, 575-576.

[8]   MacGillivray, L. R. & Atwood, J. L. (1999). Structural classification and general principles for the design of spherical molecular hosts. *Angew. Chem., Int. Ed.*, 38, 1018-1033.

[9]   Leininger, S., Olenyuk, B. & Stang, P. J. (2000). Self-assembly of discrete cyclic nanostructures mediated by transition metals. *Chem. Rev.*, 100, 853-908.

[10] D'Arcy W. Thompson (1992). *On Growth and Form*. Cambridge: Cambridge University Press.

[11] Caspar, D. L. D. & Klug, A. (1962). Physical principles in the construction of regular viruses. *Cold Spring Harb. Symp. Quant. Biol.*, 27, 1-24.

[12] Stagg, S. M., Gürkan, C., Fowler, D. M., LaPointe, P., Foss, T. R., Potter, C. S., Carragher, B. & Balch, W. E. (2006). Structure of the Sec13/31 COPII coat cage. *Nature*, 439, 234-238.

[13] Coulibaly, F., Chiu, E., Ikeda, K., Gutmann, S., Haebel, P. W., Schulze-Briese, C., Mori, H. & Metcalf, P. (2007). The molecular organization of cypovirus polyhedra. *Nature*, 446, 97-101.

[14] Fotin, A., Cheng, Y., Sliz, P., Grigorieff, N., Harrison, S. C., Kirchhausen, T., Walz, T. (2004). Molecular model for a complete clathrin lattice from electron cryomicroscopy. *Nature*, 432, 573-579.

[15] Duda, R. L. (1998). Protein chainmail: catenated protein in viral capsids. *Cell*, 94, 55-60.

[16] Wikoff, W. R., Liljas, L., Duda, R. L., Tsuruta, H., Hendrix, R. W. & Johnson, J. E. (2000). Topologically linked protein rings in the bacteriophage HK97 capsid. *Science*, 289, 2129-2133.

[17] Seeman, N. C. (2003). DNA in a material world. *Nature*, 421, 427-431.

[18] Seeman, N. C. (2005). Nucleic acid nanostructures: bottom-up control of geometry on the nanoscale. *Rep. Prog. Phys.*, 68, 237-270.

[19] Seeman, N. C. (2004). Nanotechnology and the double helix. *Sci. Am.*, 290, 64-75.

[20] Seeman, N. C. (1982). Nucleic acid junctions and lattices. *J. Theor. Biol.*, 99, 237-247.

[21] Aldaye, F. A., Palmer, A. L. & Sleiman, H. F. (2008). Assembling materials with DNA as the guide. *Science*, 321, 1795-1799.

[22] Heckel, A. & Famulok, M. (2008). Building objects from nucleic acids for a nanometer world. *Biochimie*, 90, 1096-1107.

[23] Simmel, F. C. (2008). Three-dimensional nanoconstruction with DNA. *Angew. Chem., Int. Ed.*, 47, 5884-5887.

[24] Lin, C., Liu, Y. & Yan, H. (2009). Designer DNA nanoarchitectures. *Biochemistry*, 48, 1663-1674.

[25] Zhang, C., He, Y., Su, M., Ko, S. H., Ye, T., Leng, Y., Sun, X., Ribbe, A. E., Jiang, W. & Mao, C. (2009). DNA self-assembly: from 2D to 3D. *Faraday Discuss.*, 143, 1-13.

[26] Adleman, L. M. (1994). Molecular computation of solutions to combinatorial problems. *Science*, 266, 1021-1024.

[27] Jonoska, N., Karl, S. A. & Saito, M. (1999). Three dimensional DNA structures in computing. *BioSystems*, 52, 143-153.

[28] LaVan, D. A., McGuire, T. & Langer, R. (2003). Small-scale systems for in vivo drug delivery. *Nat. Biotechnol.*, 21, 1184-1191.

[29] Erben, C. M., Goodman, R. P. & Turberfield, A. J. (2006). Single-molecule protein encapsulation in a rigid DNA cage. *Angew. Chem., Int. Ed.*, 45, 7414-7417.

[30] Bath, J. & Turberfield, A. J. (2007). DNA nanomachines. *Nat. Nanotechnol.*, 2, 275-284.

[31] Goodman, R. P., Heilemann, M., Doose, S., Erben, C. M., Kapanidis, A. N. & Turberfield, A. J. (2008). Reconfigurable, braced, three-dimensional DNA nanostructures. *Nat. Nanotechnol.*, 3, 93-96.

[32] Mitchell, N., Schlapak, R., Kastner, M., Armitage, D., Chrzanowski, W., Riener, J., Hinterdorfer, P., Ebner, A. & Howorka, S. (2009). A DNA nanostructure for the functional assembly of chemical groups with tunable stoichiometry and defined nanoscale geometry. *Angew. Chem., Int. Ed.*, 48, 525-527.

[33] Zhang, C. & Mao, C. (2008). DNA Nanotechnology: Bacteria as factories. *Nat. Nanotechnol.*, 3, 707-708.

[34] Qiu, W.-Y. & Zhai, X.-D. (2005). Molecular design of Goldberg polyhedral links. *J. Mol. Struct. THEOCHEM*, 756, 163-166.

[35] Starck, M. (2007). *A Ride Through the Polyhedra World*. http://www.ac-noumea.nc/maths/polyhedr/index_.htm.

[36] Alvarez, S. (2005). Polyhedra in (inorganic) chemistry. *Dalton Trans.*, 2005, 2209-2233.

[37] Goldberg, M. (1937). A class of multi-symmetryic polyhedra. *Tohoku Math. J.*, 43, 104-108.

[38] Kroto, H. W., Health, J. R., O'Brien, S. C., Curl, R. F. & Smalley, R. E. (1985). C_{60}: buckminsterfullerene. *Nature*, 318, 162-163.

[39] Fowler, P. W. & Manolopoulos, D. E. (2007). *An Atlas of Fullerenes*. Dover: Dover Publications.

[40] Johnson, J. E. & Speir, J. A. (1997). Quasi-equivalent viruses: a paradigm for protein assemblies. *J. Mol. Biol.*, 269, 665-675.

[41] Watson, J. D. & Crick, F. H. C. (1953). A structure for deoxyribose nucleic acid. *Nature*, 171, 737-738.

[42] Watson, J. D. & Crick, F. H. C. (1953). Genetical implications of the structure of deoxyribonucleic acid. *Nature*, 171, 964-967.

[43] Hagerman, P. J. (1988). Flexibility of DNA. *Annu. Rev. Biophys Biomol. Struct.*, 17, 265-286.

[44] Qiu, H., Dewan, J. C. & Seeman N. C. (1997). A DNA decamer with a sticky end: the crystal structure of d-CGACGATCGT. *J. Mol. Biol.*, 267, 881-898.

[45] Dickerson, R. E. (1982). The anatomy of A-, B-, and Z-DNA. *Science,* 216, 475-485.
[46] Seeman, N. C. & Kallenbach, N. R. (1994). DNA Branched Junctions. *Annu. Rev. Biophys. Biomol. Struct.,* 23, 53-86.
[47] Seeman, N. C. & Kallenbach, N. R. (1983). Design of immobile nucleic acid junctions. *Biophys. J.,* 44, 201-209.
[48] Broker, T. R. & Lehman, I. R. (1971). Branched DNA molecules: intermediates in T4 recombination. *J. Mol. Biol.,* 60, 131-149.
[49] Wang, Y., Mueller, J. E., Kemper, B. & Seeman, N. C. (1991). Assembly and characterization of five-arm and six-arm DNA branched junctions. *Biochemistry,* 30, 5667-5674.
[50] Wang, X. & Seeman, N. C. (2007). Assembly and Characterization of 8-Arm and 12-Arm DNA Branched Junctions. *J. Am. Chem. Soc.,* 129, 8169-8176.
[51] Chen, J. & Seeman, N. C. (1991). Synthesis from DNA of a molecule with the connectivity of a cube. *Nature,* 350, 631-633.
[52] Zhang, Y. & Seeman, N. C. (1994). Construction of a DNA-truncated octahedron. *J. Am. Chem. Soc.,* 116, 1661-1669.
[53] Goodman, R. P., Berry, R. M. & Turberfield, A. J. (2004). The single-step synthesis of a DNA tetrahedron. *Chem. Commun.,* 12, 1372-1373.
[54] Goodman, R. P., Schaap, I. A. T., Tardin, C. F., Erben, C. M., Berry, R. M., Schmidt, C. F., Turberfield, A. J. (2005). Rapid Chiral Assembly of Rigid DNA Building Blocks for Molecular Nanofabrication. *Science,* 310, 1661-1665.
[55] He, Y., Ye, T., Su, M., Zhang, C., Ribbe, A. E., Jiang, W. & Mao, C. (2008). Hierarchical self-assembly of DNA into symmetric supramolecular polyhedra. *Nature,* 452, 198-201.
[56] Ke, Y., Sharma, J., Liu, M., Jahn, K., Liu, Y. & Yan, H. (2009). Scaffolded DNA origami of a DNA tetrahedron molecular container. *Nano Lett.,* 9, 2445-2447.
[57] Li, Z., Wei, B., Nangreave, J., Lin, C., Liu, Y., Mi, Y., & Yan, H. (2009). A replicable tetrahedral nanostructure self-assembled from a single DNA strand, *J. Am. Chem. Soc., 131,* 13093–13098.
[58] Mastroianni, A. J., Claridge, S. A. & Alivisatos, A. P. (2009). Pyramidal and chiral groupings of gold nanocrystals assembled using DNA scaffolds. *J. Am. Chem. Soc.,* 131, 8455-8459.
[59] Özhalıcı-Ünal, H. & Armitage, B. A. (2009). Fluorescent DNA nanotags based on a self-assembled DNA tetrahedron. *ACS Nano.,* 3, 425-433.

[60] Kato, T., Goodman, R. P., Erben, C. M., Turberfield, A. J. & Namba, K. (2009). High-resolution structural analysis of a DNA nanostructure by cryoEM. *Nano Lett.*, 9, 2747-2750.

[61] He, Y. & Mao, C. (2006). Balancing flexibility and stress in DNA nanostructures. *Chem. Commun.*, 9, 968-969.

[62] He, Y., Chen, Y., Liu, H. P., Ribbe, A. E. & Mao, C. (2005). Self-Assembly of Hexagonal DNA Two-Dimensional (2D) Arrays. *J. Am. Chem. Soc.*, 127, 12202-12203.

[63] Yan, H., Park, S. H., Finkelstein, G., Reif, J. H. & LaBean, T. H. (2003). DNA-Templated Self-Assembly of Protein Arrays and Highly Conductive Nanowires. *Science*, 301, 1882-1884.

[64] He, Y., Tian, Y., Chen, Y., Deng, Z., Ribbe, A. E. & Mao, C. (2005). Sequence Symmetry as a Tool for Designing DNA Nanostructures. *Angew. Chem., Int. Ed.*, 44, 6694-6696.

[65] He, Y., Tian, Y., Ribbe, A. E. & Mao, C. (2006). Highly Connected Two-Dimensional Crystals of DNA Six-Point-Stars. *J. Am. Chem. Soc.*, 128, 15978-15979.

[66] Li, X., Yang, X., Qi, J. & Seeman, N. C. (1996). Antiparallel DNA Double Crossover Molecules As Components for Nanoconstruction. *J. Am. Chem. Soc.*, 118, 6131-6140.

[67] Sa-Ardyen, P., Vologodskii, A. V. & Seeman, N. C. (2003). The Flexibility of DNA Double Crossover Molecules. *Biophys. J.*, 84, 3829-3837.

[68] Qiu, W.-Y. (2000). Knot theory, DNA topology, and molecular symmetry breaking. In: D. Bonchev & D. H. Rouvray (Eds.), Chemical topology—applications and techniques, Mathematical Chemistry Series (Vol. 6, pp. 175-237). Amsterdam: Gordon and Breach Science Publishers.

[69] Zhang, C., Ko, S. H., Su, M., Leng, Y., Ribbe, A. E., Jiang, W. & Mao, C. (2009). Symmetry Controls the Face Geometry of DNA Polyhedra. *J. Am. Chem. Soc.*, 131, 1413-1315.

[70] Andersen, E. S., Dong, M., Nielsen, M. M., Jahn, K., Subramani, R., Mamdouh, W., Golas, M. M., Sander, B., Stark, H., Oliveira, C. L. P., Pedersen, J. S., Birkedal, V., Besenbacher, F., Gothelf, K. V. & Kjems, J. (2009). Self-assembly of a nanoscale DNA box with a controllable lid. *Nature*, 459, 73-76.

[71] Kuzuya, A. & Komiyama, M. (2009). Design and construction of a box-shaped 3D-DNA origami. *Chem. Commun.*, 28, 4182-4184.

[72] Frisch, H. L. & Wasserman, E. (1961). Chemical Topology. *J. Am. Chem. Soc.*, 83, 3789-3795.

[73] Shih, W. M., Quispe, J. D. & Joyce, G. F. (2004). A 1.7-kilobase single-stranded DNA that folds into a nanoscale octahedron. *Nature*, 427, 618-621.

[74] Andersen, F. F., Knudsen, B., Oliveira, C. L. P., Frøhlich, R. F., Krüger, D., Bungert, J., Agbandje-McKenna, M., McKenna, R., Juul, S., Veigaard, C., Koch, J., Rubinstein, J. L., Guldbrandtsen, B., Hede, M. S., Karlsson, G., Andersen, A. H., Pedersen, J. S. & Knudsen, B. R. (2008). Assembly and structural analysis of a covalently closed nanoscale DNA cage. *Nucleic Acids Res.*, 36, 1113-1119.

[75] Oliveira, C. L. P., Juul, S., Jørgensen, H. L., Knudsen, B., Tordrup, D., Oteri, F., Falconi, M., Koch, J., Desideri, A., Pedersen, J. S., Andersen, F. F. & Knudsen, B. R.(2010) . Structure of nanoscale truncated octahedral DNA cages: Variation of single-stranded linker regions and influence on assembly yields. *ACS Nano.*, DOI: 0.1021/nn901510v.

[76] He, Y., Su, M., Fang, P., Zhang, C., Ribbe, A. E., Jiang, W., & Mao, C. (2010). On the chirality of self-assembled DNA octahedral. *Angew. Chem., Int. Ed.*, *49*, 748-751.

[77] Zhang, X., Yan, H., Shen, Z. & Seeman, N. C. (2002). Paranemic cohesion of topologically-closed DNA molecules. *J. Am. Chem. Soc.*, 124, 12940-12941.

[78] Rothemund, P. W. K. (2006). Scaffolded DNA origami: from generalized multicrossovers to polygonal networks. In J. H. Chen, N. Jonoska & G. Rozenberg (Eds.), Nanotechnology: science and computation (pp. 3-21). Heidelberg: Springer.

[79] Seeman, N. C. (1998). Nucleic acid nanostructures and topology. *Angew. Chem., Int. Ed.*, 37, 3220-3238.

[80] Zimmermann, J., Cebulla, M. P. J., Mönninghoff, S. & von Kiedrowski, G. (2008). Self-assembly of a DNA dodecahedron from 20 trisoligonucleotides with C_{3h} linkers. *Angew. Chem., Int. Ed.*, 47, 3626-3630.

[81] Chandra, M., Keller, S., Gloeckner, C., Bornemann, B. & Marx, A. (2007). New branched DNA constructs. *Chem. Eur. J.*, 1?, 3558-3564.

[82] Scheffler, M., Dorenbeck, A., Jordan, S., Wüstefeld, M. & von Kiedrowski, G. (1999). Self-assembly of trisoligonucleotidyls: the case for nano-acetylene and nano-cyclobutadiene. *Angew. Chem., Int. Ed.*, 38, 3311-3315.

[83] Eckardt, L. H., Naumann, K., Pankau, W. M., Rein, M., Schweitzer, M., Windhab, N. & von Kiedrowski, G. (2002). DNA nanotechnology: chemical copying of connectivity. *Nature*, 420, 286-286.

[84] Zhang, C., Su, M., He, Y., Zhao, X., Fang, P., Ribbe, A. E., Jiang, W. & Mao, C. (2008). Conformational flexibility facilitates self-assembly of complex DNA nanostructures. *Proc. Natl. Acad. Sci. U. S. A.*, 105, 10665-10669.

[85] Douglas, S. M., Dietz, H., Liedl, T., Högberg, B., Graf, F. & Shih, W. M. (2009). Self-assembly of DNA into nanoscale three-dimensional shapes. *Nature*, 459, 414-418.

[86] Bhatia, D., Mehtab, S., Krishnan, R., Indi, S. S., Basu, A. & Krishnan, Y. (2009). Icosahedral DNA nanocapsules by modular assembly. *Angew. Chem., Int. Ed.*, 48, 4134-4137.

[87] Aldaye, F. A. & Sleiman, H. F. (2007). Modular access to structurally switchable 3D discrete DNA assemblies. *J. Am. Chem. Soc.*, 129, 13376-13377.

[88] Erben, C. M., Goodman, R. P. & Turberfield, A. J. (2007). A self-assembled DNA bipyramid. *J. Am. Chem. Soc.*, 129, 6992-6993.

[89] Rakotondradany, F., Sleiman, H. F. & Whitehead, M. A. (2007). Theoretical study of self-assembled hydrogen-bonded azodibenzoic acid tapes and rosettes. *J. Mol. Struct. THEOCHEM*, 806, 39-50.

[90] Aldaye, F. A. & Sleiman, H. F. (2007). Dynamic DNA templates for discrete gold nanoparticle assemblies: control of geometry, modularity, write/erase and structural switching. *J. Am. Chem. Soc.*, 129, 4130-4131.

[91] Qiu, W.-Y., Zhai, X.-D. & Qiu, Y.-Y. (2008). Architecture of Platonic and Archimedean polyhedral links. *Sci. China Ser. B-Chem.*, 51, 13-18.

[92] Seife, C. (2003). Polyhedral model gives the universe an unexpected twist. *Science*, 302, 209-210.

[93] Adams, C. C. (1994). The Knot Book-an Elementary Introduction to the Mathematical Theory of Knots. New York: W. H. Freeman and Company.

[94] Cromwell, P. R. (2004). *Knots and Links*. Cambridge: Cambridge University Press.

[95] Jablan, S. & Sazdanovic, R. (2008). *Linknot: Knot Theory by Computer*. Singapore: World Scientific.

[96] Hu, G., Zhai, X.-D., Lu, D. & Qiu, W.-Y., (2008). The architecture of Platonic polyhedral links. *J. Math. Chem.*, 46, 592-602.

[97] Lu, D., Hu, G., Qiu, Y.-Y. & Qiu, W.-Y. (2010). Topological transformation of dual polyhedral links. *MATCH Commun. Math. Comput. Chem.*, 63, 67-78.

[98] Lu, D. & Qiu, W.-Y. (2010). The keeping and reversal of chirality for dual links. *MATCH Commun. Math. Comput. Chem.*, 63, 79-90.

[99] Walba, D. M. (1985). Topological stereochemistry. *Tetrahedron*, 41, 3161-3212.

[100] Sumners, D. W. (1987). The knot theory of molecules. *J. Math. Chem.*, 1, 1-14.

[101] In geometry, Schlegel diagram remains all topological properties, such as vertex degree and connections, while represents three dimensional graph in two dimensional planes. More about Schlegel diagram see ref. [1].

[102] Archdeacon, D., Siran, J. & Skoviera, M. (1992). Self-dual regular maps from medial graphs. *Acta Math. Univ. Comenianae*, 61, 57-64.

[103] Flapan, E. (1998). Topological rubber gloves *J. Math. Chem.*, 23, 31-49.

[104] Flapan, E. (2000). When Topology Meets Chemistry: a Topological Look at Molecular Chirality. Cambridge: Cambridge University Press.

[105] Qiu, W.-Y. & Xin, H.-W. (1997). Molecular design and topological chirality of the Tq-Möbius ladders. *J. Mol. Struct. THEOCHEM*, 401, 151-156.

[106] Qiu, W.-Y. & Xin, H.-W. (1997). Molecular design and tailor of the doubled knots. *J. Mol. Struct. THEOCHEM*, 397, 33-37.

[107] Qiu, W.-Y. & Xin, H.-W. (1998). Topological structure of closed circular DNA. *J. Mol. Struct. THEOCHEM*, 428, 35-39.

[108] Qiu, W.-Y. & Xin, H.-W. (1998). Topological chirality and achirality of DNA knots. *J. Mol. Struct. THEOCHEM*, 429, 81-86.

[109] Mislow, K. (1996). A commetary on the topological chirality and achirality of molecules. *Croat. Chem. Acta.*, 69, 485-511.

[110] Simon, J. (1986). Topological chirality of certain molecules. *Topology*, 25, 229-235.

[111] Liang, C. Z. & Mislow, K. (1994). On amphicheiral knots. *J. Math. Chem.*, 15, 1-34.

[112] Liang, C. Z. & Mislow, K. (1994). A left-right classification of topologically chiral knots. *J. Math. Chem.*, 15, 35-62.

[113] Liang, C. Z. & Mislow, K. (1994). Classification of topologically chiral molecules. *J. Math. Chem.*, 15, 245-260.

[114] Liang, C. Z. & Mislow, K. (1995). Topological chirality and achirality of links. *J. Math. Chem.*, 18, 1-24.

[115] Cheng, X.-S., Qiu, W.-Y. & Zhang, H.-P. (2009). A novel molecular design of polyhedral links and their chiral analysis. *MATCH Commun. Math. Comput. Chem.*, 62, 115-130.

[116] Hu, G. & Qiu, W.-Y. (2008). Extended Goldberg polyhedra. *MATCH Commun. Math. Comput. Chem.*, 59, 585-594.

[117] Hu, G., Qiu, W.-Y. (2009). Extended Goldberg polyhedral links with even tangles. *MATCH Commun. Math. Comput. Chem.*, 61, 737-752.

[118] Hu, G. & Qiu, W.-Y. (2009). Extended Goldberg polyhedral links with odd tangles. *MATCH Commun. Math. Comput. Chem.*, 61, 753-766.

[119] In fact, the calculation of the number of component rings of Extended Goldberg polyhedra when k is odd is mathematically equivalent to the problem of central circuits counting of 4-valent graphs. However, until now, it still remains unsolved. More about central circuits counting problem on 4-valent graphs see ref. [120-122]

[120] Deza, M., Huang, T. & Lih, K.-O. (2002). Central circuit coverings of octahedrites and medial polyhedra. *J. Math. Res. Exposition*, 22, 49-65.

[121] Dutour, M. & Deza, M. (2004). Goldberg-Coxeter construction for 3- and 4-valent plane graphs. *Electron. J. Combinatorics*, 11, R20.

[122] Deza, M. & Dutour, M. (2005). Zigzag structure of simple bifaced polyhedra. *Combinatorics, Probability Comput.*, 14, 31-57.

[123] Jonoska, N. & Twarock, R. (2008). Blueprints for dodecahedral DNA cages. *J. Phys. A: Math. Theor.*, 41, 304043-304057.

[124] Grayson, N. E., Taorminab, A. & Twarock, R., (2009). DNA duplex cage structures with icosahedral symmetry. *Theor. Comput. Sci.* 410, 1440-1447.

[125] Jonoska, N. & Saito, M. (2002). Boundary Components of Thickened Graphs. In: N. Jonoska & N. C. Seeman (Eds.), Lecture notes in computer science: DNA7 (Vol. 2340, pp. 70-81). London: Springer-Verlag.

[126] Tang, L., Johnson, K. N., Ball, L. A., Lin, T., Yeager, M. & Johnson, J. E. (2001). The structure of Pariacoto virus reveals a dodecahedral cage of duplex RNA. *Nat. Struct. Mol. Biol.*, 8, 77-83.

[127] Rudnick, J. & Bruinsma, R. (2005). Icosahedral packing of RNA viral genomes. *Phys. Rev. Lett.*, 94, 038101-038105.

[128] Andersson, S. (2008). The structure of virus capsids. *Z. Anorg. Allg. Chem.*, 634, 2161-2170.

[129] Andersson, S. (2008). Description of virus capsid structures with methods from inorganic solid. *Z.Anorg. Allg. Chem.*, 634, 2504-2510.

[130] Andersson, S. (2009). Virus evolution and the beginning. *Z. Anorg. Allg. Chem.*, 635, 717-724.

[131] Andersson, S. (2009). Virus structures, stellations, spikes, and rods. *Z. Anorg. Allg. Chem.*, 635, 725-731.

[132] Andersson,S. (2008). *Intrinsic Structure of Virus Capsids.* Sweden: Sandforsk.

[133] Yang, Y.-M. & Qiu, W.-Y. (2007). Molecular design and mathematical analysis of carbon nanotube links. *MATCH Commun. Math. Comput. Chem.*, 58, 635-646.

[134] Hu, G. & Qiu, W.-Y. (2010). Two Combinatorial Operations and a Knot Theoretical Approach for Fullerene Polyhedra . *MATCH Commun. Math. Comput. Chem.*, 63, 347-362.

[135] Cheng, X. S., Liu, S. Y., Zhang, H. & Qiu ,W.-Y.(2010). Fabrication of a Family of Pyramidal Links and Their Genus, *MATCH Commun. Math. Comput. Chem.*, 63, 623-636.

[136] Cheng, X. S., Zhang, H., Hu, G. & Qiu, W.-Y.(2010). The Architecture and Jones Polynomials of Cycle–crossover Polyhedral Links, *MATCH Commun. Math. Comput. Chem.*, 63, 637-656.

[137] National Research Council. (1995). *Commission on Physical Sciences, Mathematics, and Applications.* Washington, D. C.: National Academy Press.

[138] Torquato, S., Jiao, Y. (2009). Dense packings of the Platonic and Archimedean solids. *Nature*, 460, 876-879.

INDEX

A

acetylene, 56
achievement, 10, 26
acid, 52, 53, 54, 56, 57
Adams, 57
aesthetics, 11
AFM, 23, 27
air, 3
algorithm, 45
Amsterdam, 55
anatomy, 54
annealing, 8, 17, 21, 22, 29
artistic, 1
asymmetry, 5, 22, 47
Atlas, 53

B

background information, 2
bacteriophage, 52
base pair, 22
benefits, 4, 15
binding, 23
biomacromolecules, 4, 41, 43, 47
biomolecular, 34
biotechnology, 4
blocks, 10
bottom-up, 52
building blocks, 10

C

carbon, 3, 60
chemical structures, 3
China, 49, 57
chiral, 19, 39, 41, 43, 54, 58, 59
chiral group, 54
chiral molecules, 58
chirality, vii, 24, 34, 39, 41, 47, 56, 58
classes, 39, 43
classification, 3, 36, 39, 51, 58
coherence, 26
cohesion, 4, 5, 56
colors, 9, 11, 30, 37, 38
complement, 8
complementarity, 29
complementary DNA, 20
complexity, 1, 22
computation, 45, 47, 52, 56
computer science, 59
computing, 52
concentration, 10, 13, 14, 15, 21, 27
concrete, 11
configuration, 4, 9, 25
Congress, iv
connectivity, 16, 54, 57
construction, vii, 5, 11, 15, 17, 25, 28, 31, 33, 37, 41, 51, 55, 59
control, 5, 9, 15, 25, 52, 57

voiding, 10